Hello Gorgeous

Hello 70

How to Stay Younger Longer

By

Helen Gibson-Nicholas

DISCLAIMER

The information in this book is not offered to treat, cure, or diagnose any disease or chronic health problem. It is not meant to replace a one-to-one consultation with a physician.

The author of this book has provided this information for personal and informational purposes only. It is not meant to be construed as an attempt to practice medicine or offer a cure for any chronic health condition.

The author of this book has tried to offer current and accurate information and makes no warranties, representations, or assurances as to the accuracy, currency, or completeness of the information provided.

The author of this book shall not be liable for any damages or injury resulting from your access to, or inability to access, this book, or from your reliance upon any information provided in this book.

DEDICATION

This book is dedicated to my children and my grandchildren.

Find your light and light up your part of the world.

ACKNOWLEDGMENTS

I must thank my patient, kind, helpful, genius husband. Without him, this book would not have been possible.

I would like to thank Joshua Rosenthal and The Institute of Integrative Nutrition for giving me the knowledge that inspired this book.

I lovingly thank my Heavenly Father for never giving up on me.

ABOUT HELEN

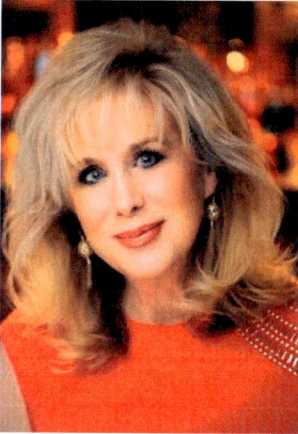

Helen Gibson-Nicholas is a health and beauty expert and her career has extended over thirty years. She is an integrative nutrition health coach, certified image consultant, master barber- cosmetologist, and professional makeup artist. Helen is also a radio talk show host, author, and public speaker. Often referred to as The Total Image Coach, she has performed more than 12,000 makeovers to help women and men find their gorgeous potential.

She believes that finding your most flattering hairstyle, clothing, makeup colors and makeup techniques reveal the confidence in the real you and gets you noticed. She calls this the gorgeous potential. Her motto is: "I help you look like who you want to become." Her passion is health and beauty from the inside out, though, teaching others about the importance of healthy choices for your diet, your soul, and your spirit.

Helen is founder and owner of Hello Gorgeous Cosmetics and Hello Gorgeous Salon and Spa in Fairview, TX. Hello Gorgeous Salon and Spa specializes in anti-aging facials, makeovers, bridal services, and hair design. When Helen founded Hello Gorgeous Cosmetics in 1987, her goal was to make an affordable anti-aging skin care system that was not chemically laden with unsafe and carcinogenic ingredients.

Her aloe skin care has been free of paraben, dye, sulfate, propylene glycol, phthalates, BHT, DMDM hydantoin, triethanolamine and other chemicals considered toxic or unsafe for human use since the 1980s. In fact, her products were green before green became the buzz word for pure, natural, and environmentally safe products.

Helen, who is 70, has consistently been an example of how to age beautifully and successfully.

Learn more about Helen, anti-aging news, and products at the following websites.

Skin care and makeup at:

HelloGorgeous.com

Beauty tips at:

BoomerBeautyBlog.com

Health news at:

WholelifeNutrition.me

Clean crafted wines:

HelloGorgeous.wine

About hello gorgeous

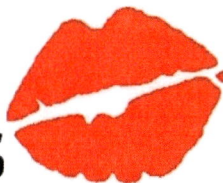

When I finish with my client and say: "Hello Gorgeous," a big smile beams from their face as they peer into the mirror to see the finished result of their makeover. Hello, my name is Helen Gibson-Nicholas. I love making women smile. At a very young age I knew that I was supposed to help women gain more confidence through success with their image. I started doing 'comb-outs' for my mother and her friends at the age of fourteen in the early sixties. This evolved into doing makeup on them also.

I loved the makeup and clothing of the sixties, which is now considered the most fashionable decade of them all. It was all about big-and-bold looks like fake lashes, dramatic cat eyes, and painted-on bottom lashes. Short bobs, bangs, and mini-skirts reigned. Moving into the seventies, short bobs grew into layered shags which ultimately produced the famous Charlie's Angels look. Cat eyes and lumpy mascara of the sixties turned into yummy shadows for disco glam and sun kissed neutrals for the emerging California-girl glow.

My favorite decade has to be the eighties where "more is more" perfectly describes it. Everyone let their pencil thin brows grow back with a vengeance. Blue eye shadow, dark lip liner, and loads of blush ruled. Big hair and shoulder pads equaled smaller hips for everyone. The nineties brought us heavy black eyeliner, plucked-to-death brows, nude cheeks and mocha lipstick. Top-of-the-head ponies reigned, tamed afros were gelled and curled, and zig-zag hair parts were introduced.

The new millennium brought us acrylic glittery nails, fake tans, chunky highlights, hair extensions, thick eyeliner and frosted lips.

This may be a decade to forget. Moving forward, leaving the glitz and gloss behind, mineral makeup was introduced. It is my favorite because it puts a natural, magic coating over the skin that reflects light and minimizes flaws. Highlights turned into ombres or balayage which graduate hair color from dark to light and visa-versa.

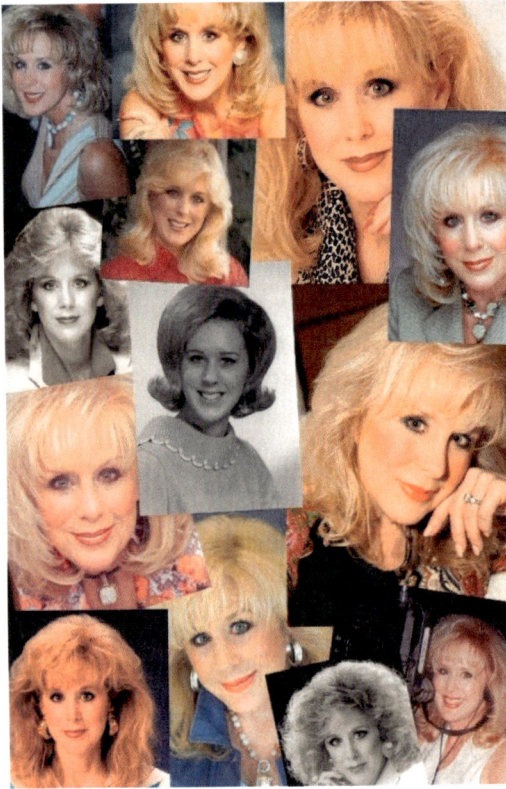

Now facial contouring rages with the makeup perfectionists but be careful, you could end up looking like a striped bass! Brows are back with even more vengeance and flat ironing is evolving into simple soft waves. Long hair reigns. Mineral makeup glows in all the right places and matt lips with glitter star at special occasions. I've been there through it all. The collage is a collection of pictures that span over fifty years (ages eighteen to sixty-nine).

I do love to help women find their 'gorgeous potential,' but I also have a passion for anti-aging! Just what is a 70-year-old grandma supposed to look like anyway? Maybe it's just the baby boomer in me, but I don't want to grow up if I have to give up.

That's why I started making my own skin care over thirty years ago with NO parabens, artificial colors, fragrances and unnecessary chemicals like propylene glycol (instead of plant-derived glycerin). Of course, our famous double aloe base (instead of water) is the secret to youth. It does three things water can't do:

1) it penetrates the dermis, 2) it is a carrier agent delivering other key nutrient factors, and 3) it stimulates collagen production up to eight times faster than normal. Yes, I do believe I have discovered the Fountain of Youth!

My clients say, "I want to look like you when I grow up!" That is why I am writing this book. I am in the skin care business, so obviously, I believe that you must have a religious skin care regimen with natural, wholesome ingredients. My program, *Ten Minutes A Day, Keeps The Wrinkles Away,* works because of the holistic combination of real ingredients!

As an Integrative Nutrition Health Coach, I also know there is more to anti-aging than just rubbing creams and serums on your face or getting plastic surgery. At the age of forty, I faced a serious health problem. I could not understand why I was so sick. I didn't smoke, drink, or chew! ☺ That is when my journey to understand health and nutrition began. I have spent the last thirty years researching and speaking on this topic. I received a fabulous education at the Institute of Integrative Nutrition in New York. I want to share this valuable information with you. It could save your life. I know it will help you stay younger longer.

I hope you love my new book, *Hello Gorgeous Hello 70!*

FIRST THOUGHTS
STAY YOUNGER LONGER

Jules Renard said: "It's not how old you are, it's how you are old."

DID YOU KNOW?

One out of five people is over sixty-five, and potentially over one million are Centenarians. Ten thousand people turn sixty-five every day! In 2029 over seventy million will be over the age of sixty-five and by 2030, eighty million will be on Medicare. Most of these people are Baby Boomers, born between 1946 and 1964.

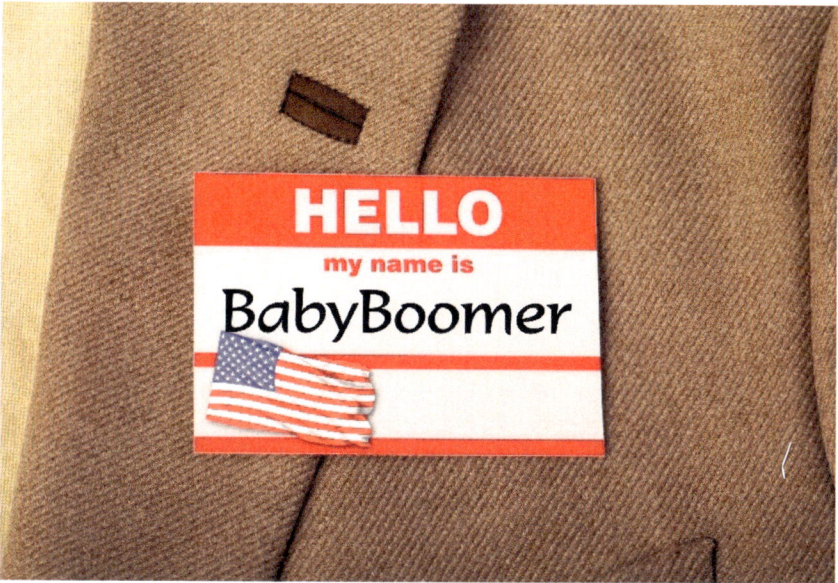

There were more babies born during that time than at any other time in history. Baby Boomers make up forty percent of the population and control eighty percent of personal financial assets and more than half of all consumers spending.

You may not be a Centenarian or a Baby Boomer but you are aging! The average life expectancy in the United States is 76 for males and 81 for females. These numbers only vary a little from country to country, plus or minus a couple of years.

Steve Holman, Editor of *Iron Man Magazine*, says studies show that without proper nutrients and exercise, your body will age six months extra for every year that passes after you hit forty. So, you could feel and look seventy when you are only sixty.

Some people say, "Helen, I thought you were around fifty." Of course, I appreciate the compliment, but I'm not taking any magic pills or have had a face lift. Anyone can do what I do and reverse the accelerated aging process and look and feel younger than your chronological age. For me, seventy is the new fifty!

Dermatologists, scientists, and aging experts tell us that ONLY twenty percent of skin aging is genetically determined. Fitness and nutrition experts tell us that anyone can stop and even reverse real aging. That tells me that there are things making us look and feel older than we should. So how do you want to be OLD?

In this book I will reveal SABOTAGING FACTORS to health, longevity, skin integrity, and happiness. STUFF that corrupts the aging process making you OLDER than you really should be!! STUFF doesn't have to happen.

The aging culprits I will outline in this book, all begin with the letter S. Are these S WORDS speeding up your aging process? Learn how I have STOPPED unnecessary AGING!

How do you want to be OLD? Hopefully like me, you want to live a long, happy, healthy life.

CONTENTS

Chapter 1

SADNESS

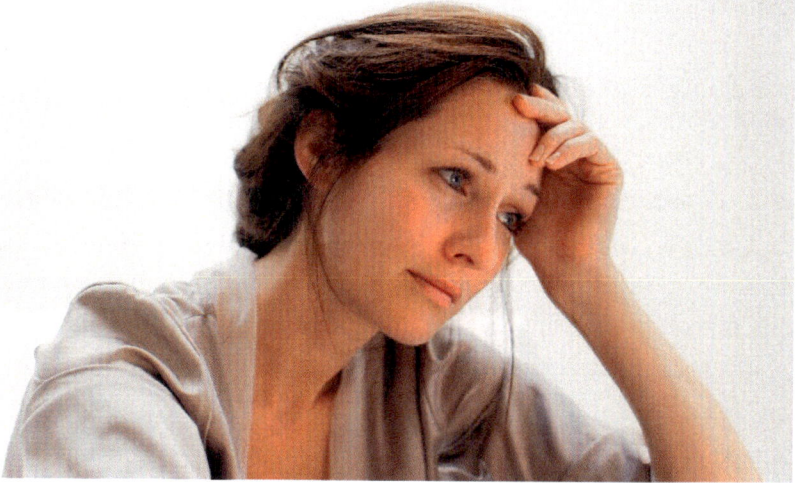

Feeling SADNESS occasionally is quite normal because 'life happens' and sometimes it is unpleasant, unkind, or unfortunate. Normally, life goes on and those unhappy days turn into happy days again. For over 350 million people around the world, SADNESS consumes them for months, even years, though. SADNESS can steal the joy of living from you and age you beyond your years.

Of course, I am talking about clinical depression or MMD (major depressive disorder). The Mayo Clinic defines depression as "a mood disorder that causes a persistent feeling of SADNESS and loss of interest." It affects how you behave, think and feel. **Depression is the leading cause of ill health and disability worldwide according to the World Health Organization (WHO) and generated 14.5 billion dollars in revenue in 2016.**

The National Institute of Mental Health reports that one of four American women ages forty to fifty are taking anti-depressants. Anti-depressants are one of the most prescribed medications in the U.S. with almost <u>300 million prescriptions per year</u>. *The Journal of the American Medical Association* (JAMA) reports the percentage of Americans taking anti-depressants almost doubled from 1999 to 2012. NBC news reported in December 2016 that one in six people were taking anti-depressants or some other psychiatric drug.

Anti-depressant drugs seem to have a unique set of SIDE EFFECTS (see that chapter for more frightening details) which include autism and ADHD (when taken during pregnancy), bone fractures, stroke, suicide, violate tendencies, emotional flatness, restlessness, sleep disturbances, and substance abuse. These drugs are not a cure and tend to add new adverse health issues on top of a serious condition.

Dr. Daniel Amen, psychiatrist and author of *Change Your Brain, Change Your Life,* said that people **"do not have a Prozac or Valium deficiency."** There are tangible reasons for depression and some may surprise you.

- A traumatic life event affects everyone differently, but remains the number one reason or cause that one withdraws from happiness and steps into SADNESS.

- Inflammation of the gastrointestinal tract is closely linked to the dysfunction of the gut-brain axis. Inflammatory cytokines interact with neural pathways known to be involved with the development of depression according to a 2012 study in *Neuropsychopharmacology.*

- SUGAR and high glycemic foods impair neuron signaling and suppress BDNF (brain derived neurotrophic factor) which is a growth hormone responsible for healthy brain neurons. Dr.

Joseph Mercola says that BDNF is critically low in both depression and schizophrenia, and animal models suggest this may even be a causative factor.

- Artificial SWEETENERS interfere with normal brain activity stimulating mood alterations and compromising emotional functioning leading to mental disorders including depression (*webMD.org*).

- Excessive electromagnetic field exposure activates VGCCs (voltage gated calcium channels) which release calcium ions that ultimately produce hydroxyl free radicals (the most destructive free radicals) that destroy cellular mitochondria. The highest density of VGCCs is in your brain. Mitochondria are responsible for cellular life and energy, without which brain cells (or any cell) cannot function properly and is now being linked to depression (*emfs.org*).

- Brain derived neurotrophic factor (BDNF) alteration genetically occurs in about twenty percent of the population which induces shrinkage of neurons in the hippocampus. A simple blood test can detect the BDNF SNP mutation that increases the risk of depression, anxiety, and memory disorders. Family heritage might be a variant, but is not the sole reason why these mental problems occur according to researchers at Weill Cornell Medical College.

Anyone suffering with this debilitating disease should seek medical attention. **Depression can cause premature aging and loss of life so it is important to examine all avenues for solutions.** Here are a few natural steps you can take for a healthier and happier life instead of just living with the dark cloud of depression or taking drugs with dreadful SIDE EFFECTS. More about that is in the SIDE EFFECTS chapter.

1. If you have had a past traumatic life event that you just can't shake off, get professional help. Facing the enemy of your peace and changing the way you react to it is one of the keys to turning around and moving forward.

   A professional advisor will help you develop a new way of assessing the event and the role it should or could play in your personal growth as opposed to depressing your future.

2. Reduce sugar, and you will reduce SADNESS. Please check out my chapter on SUGAR for even more details on how SUGAR affects your health. The link between SUGAR and depression is overwhelming. If it destroys the hormones that keep your brain healthy, why would you eat it? If it is as addictive as cocaine why would you eat it? If it is linked to heart disease and cancer, why would you eat it? SUGAR is not only aging you and making you sick, it is could be making you mentally ill with depression.

3. Exercise is good for the body and good for the brain. Many psychologists now prescribe exercise to their patients with depression. GABA (gamma aminobutyric acid) is a neurotransmitter which inhibits excessive neuronal firing. It is produced naturally when you exercise and helps to induce a state of calm. It also increases levels of serotonin, dopamine, and norepinephrine which do the same. Take a ten minute walk every day for amazing benefits.

4. Frankincense oil has been used by cultures for healing therapy for thousands of years. It was one of the three gifts of the Magi for the baby Jesus. Who knew it could help with depression? Inhaling the gentle fragrance immediately induces a feeling of calm, peace, and relaxation. It reduces heart rate and blood pressure. It influences the limbic system which is best described as the "feeling and reacting brain" through olfaction, reducing anxiety and depression.

5. Vitamin D deficiency is associated with depression. A study of seniors showed that those who were deficient in Vitamin D were eleven times more likely to be depressed. I recommend a blood test and follow with supplementation. Be sure to get sensible SUN exposure as outlined in my chapter, SUN, and produce vitamin D naturally.

6. Probiotics not only stabilize the environment of the gut, they also 'cool down' the amygdala in the brain which tends to be 'red hot' in people with depression, as reported in *gastrojournal.org*. Since depression is also found alongside gastrointestinal inflammation it is now considered a "neuropsychiatric manifestation of a chronic inflammatory syndrome," per Dr. Joseph Mercola. Eating fermented foods and probiotic supplementation can help fight off depression.

7. Omega 3 supplements with both EPA and DHA for inflammation, Coenzyme Q10 for mitochondria support, and Alpha Lipoic Acid (100 to 400 mg) to help prevent metabolic syndrome all help with preventing depression. Other nutrients that play a role in the treatment of depression are SAMe, 5-HTP, and St. John's Wort.

8. Limit EMF exposure by keeping computers, iPads, phones, etc. out of the bedroom. Get outside and back to nature whenever you can. Take walks at lunch, take more mini-vacations, eat on the patio, play golf, learn tennis, join a bird watching group, plant flowers, pull weeds, walk on the beach, or just turn your PC off.

SADNESS is affecting the way you look. I know you may have heard "it takes more muscles to frown than to smile," but it doesn't. However, there is an anti-aging caveat here. It actually takes more muscles to smile, but that is a good thing. Since your face uses more muscles to smile and usually smiles more than it frowns, it is exercising facial muscles, keeping them tight and lifted. Since those muscles are in shape, it is easier to smile than to frown, which is probably where that 'saying' came from. I'm sure you know someone who is happy and smiles a lot, and they look younger than most of their friends who don't smile as much. Now you know why.

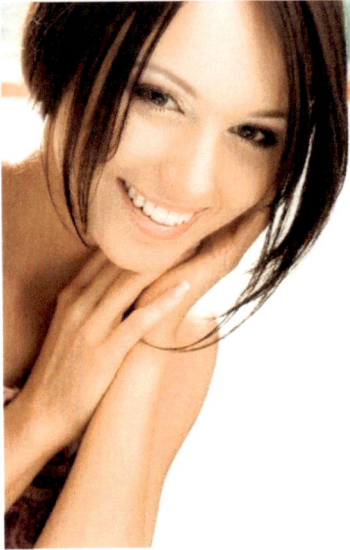

Physiognomy is the science of facial features and their effect on the brain. For our purpose here, we will discuss how your facial expressions affect your mood. The way the mind works (in layman's terms) is that it notices the patterns in your facial features and reflects that mood accordingly. When you smile, neuropeptides facilitate messaging to the whole body. Dopamine, endorphins and serotonin are released which relaxes, relieves pain, and replaces depression. So, SMILE! Studies have been done where they asked people to act sad, angry, or fearful and the same physical reactions occurred that the actual emotion would have produced: increased heart rate, sweating, elevated skin temperature, etc. Smiling in the control group produced feelings of happiness and peace. I'm not saying that smiling will cure your depression, but it will certainly make you feel better and it certainly can't hurt.

SADNESS, aka depression, is a 'dis-ease' that you can and should fight and overcome if you want to slow down the aging process and look and feel younger longer.

Get help, get healthy, and get happy!

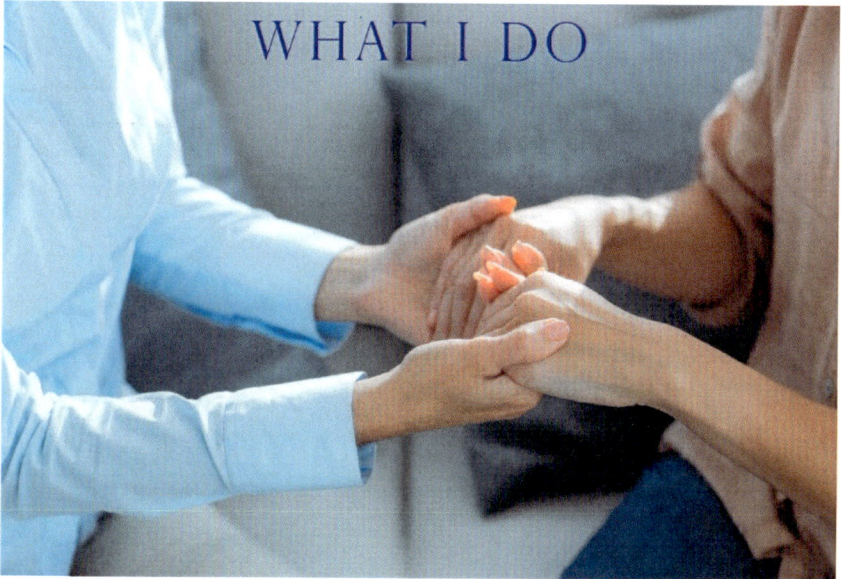

WHAT I DO

1. I have several friends who are professional counselors whom I talk to in down times.

2. Sometimes I just cry, pray, forgive, and realize that I can't control what has happened, but I can control the way I react to it.

3. I take probiotics and eat fermented foods for gut health.

4. We added an outdoor living area so that we could stay outside more.

5. I take vitamin D, omega 3, coenzyme Q10, alpha lipoic acid, and Ashwagandha/ginkgo supplements.

6. When feeling really down, I take SAMe supplements.

7. I put Frankincense in my diffuser just about every day.

8. I exercise four to five times per week.

Chapter 2

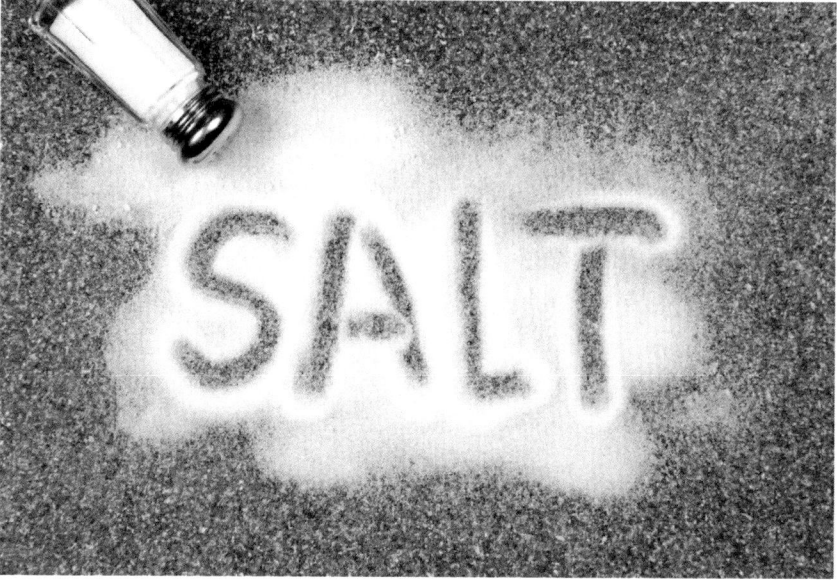

Let me tell you how this white gold became white poison. **Life is not possible without SALT, so why is it making people so sick?** The answer is that regular table SALT used today is not the original crystal SALT that our bodies need to function properly. Without SALT, you would die, but too much of the wrong salt will age you!

Unfortunately, table SALT has been 'chemically cleaned' and reduced to the combination of sodium and chloride. "Sodium chloride is an aggressive substance which is perpetually seeking a bio-chemical equalizing counterpart, so that the body's pH can remain neutral," per the book: *Water and Salt, The Essence of Life.* Your body thinks table SALT is a type of cellular poison and tries to get rid of it. We consume .4 to .7 ounces daily, but can only eliminate 0.17 ounces to 0.25. The result is overly acidic edema (excess fluid in the body tissues) which is one of the causes of cellulite. As you can see excessive sodium in your bloodstream affects the body's delicate pH balance, reducing the ability of your kidneys to remove water. This is only one of the reasons you should avoid common table salt.

Another reason is gout and rheumatism. Excess salt (only .035 ounces) requires 23 times its own cell water to neutralize. When not available, it binds with certain animal proteins to produce uric acid which deposits them directly in the bones and joints. Also, regular table SALT contains iodide (a highly toxic form of iodine) and fluoride (a greenish-yellow gas which accelerates aging). Finally, preservatives which are not required in labeling, like aluminum hydroxide which is known to prevent bridging of nervous pathways associated with Alzheimer's.

Let's explore one more major problem with SALT: HBP. High blood pressure is due to the extra fluid and extra strain on the delicate blood vessels leading to the kidneys. The imbalance of salt and water causes the heart to pump more blood that presses against the blood vessel walls greater than normal. This is hypertension and it ages you or even worse. It often goes undetected because of the lack of symptoms and is often referred to as "the silent killer."

One in three American adults (seventy-five million) has hypertension or high blood pressure. The NHLBI (National Heart, Lung, and Blood Institute) reports that about sixty-five percent of U.S. adults ages sixty and older have high blood pressure. Here are some of the potential warning signs or symptoms HBP:

- Headaches – These are common symptoms associated with many health issues, but when in doubt check your blood pressure.

- Pains in the Chest – This usually frightens everyone into the doctor's office. It could be indigestion, hypertension, or a heart attack. Hello!

- Shortness of Breath – This may happen occasionally if you are elderly or out of shape. But if it persists, get tested.

- Exhaustion – There are many reasons for this, examine the circumstances or other medical conditions. If unusual, get tested.

- Nausea and Vomiting – If not associated with something you have eaten, this is a warning not to be ignored.

- Facial Flushing – Occurs when blood vessels are dilated during high blood pressure spells.

- Ringing in the Ears – This could be the sound of impending doom.

- Lightheaded or Dizzy – When high, even slurred speech might occur.

- Nose Bleeds – Usually an advanced warning sign.

- Bloody Spots in the Eye – High blood pressure left untreated damages nerves and capillaries in this delicate area.

- Blurred Vision – Common to many health issues, but could be HBP.

- No Symptoms at All – Unfortunately that is why it is called "the silent killer."

Note: White coat syndrome is fake high blood pressure. So, take a few deep breaths and calm down before getting your blood pressure taken and take it several times. Taking your blood pressure in both arms helps rule out cardiovascular problems. It should be the same in both.

Here are a few things you can do to slow down premature aging from this potential deadly substance:

- Reduce your sugar load and don't eat table salt. Untreated sea salt or Himalayan salt is ok.

- Beet juice, garlic, and watermelon dilate blood vessels which lowers blood pressure. Other vegetables that also work are radishes, kale, celery, mustard greens, turnip greens, spinach, eggplant, leeks, scallions, string beans, and carrots.

- You can juice many of these for great results. Try one beet, a handful of kale, two carrots, two celery stalks, and a small cucumber.

- Exercise, reduce stress, and sleep seven to eight hours. Please check out the chapters SLEEPLESSNESS and STRESS for more information.

- Don't eat packaged or canned foods with added sodium.

- Basically, you must eat fresh, real food to reduce your sodium to potassium ratio.

- Learn to cook from scratch. It is so much healthier for you and your loved ones.

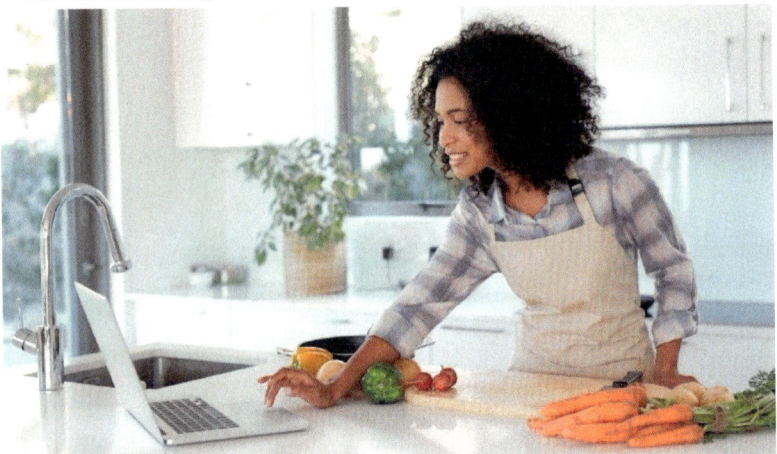

I love Himalayan salt which is in its holistic form and has naturally occurring calcium, potassium, and magnesium and numerous other minerals which enable and enhance the natural functioning of all cells. It is the best form of SALT, in my opinion. It does not affect cardio vascular issues like ordinary table SALT. For more information get the book: *Water & Life*, *The Essence of Life* by Dr. Barbara Handel and Peter Ferreira. Himalayan salt tastes delicious so you naturally use less.

If you have high blood pressure, it is aging you internally. Even your skin is affected by the bloating, toxic build-up, and lack of nutrition. The elasticity is compromised and pre-mature sagging and wrinkling shows up before it should. Do your face a favor, and don't eat table SALT.

If you want to slow down the aging process, don't eat table SALT

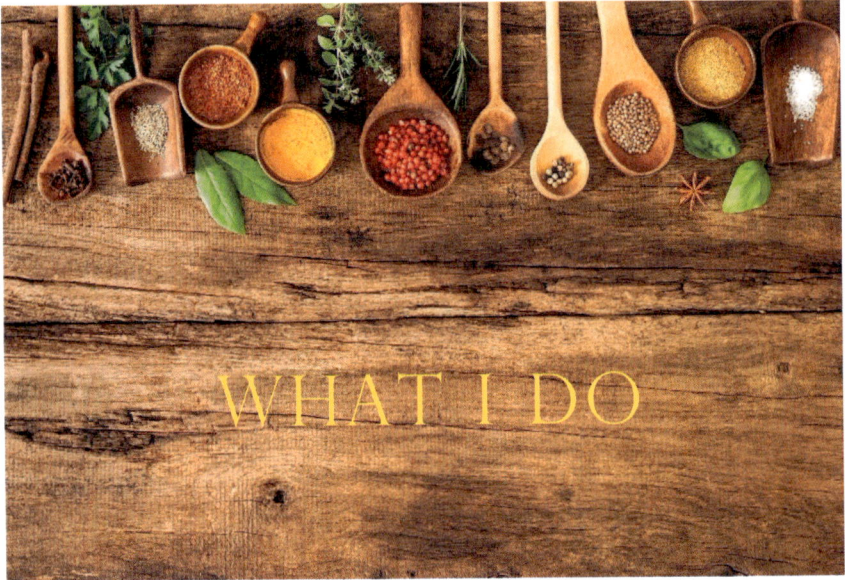

WHAT I DO

1. I always carry a little jar of Himalayan Salt in my purse.

2. I never use table salt.

3. I buy Himalayan salt in bulk from Costco. You can also now find it online and at most stores.

4. I cook from scratch and avoid packaged foods and sauces.

5. I cook with a wide variety of spices and dried herbs to add flavor and variety to meals.

6. I LOVE to juice the recipe I gave above once or twice a week.

7. Vegetables are the stars of all my meals.

Chapter 3

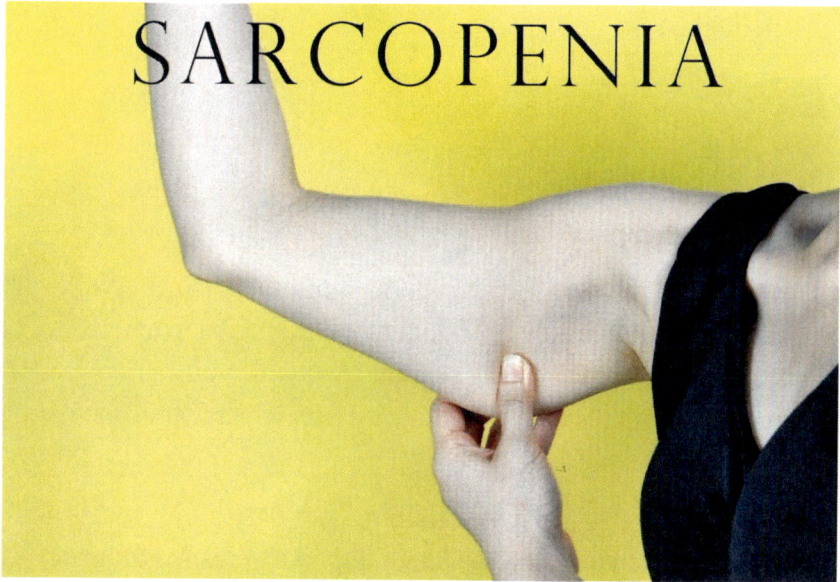

SARCOPENIA

Sarcopenia is the loss of muscle mass and function. **You lose three to five percent every decade and by age seventy, you could lose one third of your body muscle mass**. *Iron Man Magazine* reports that ninety percent of people over thirty-five lose enough muscle mass every year to burn four pounds of body fat. Losing muscle mass causes you to gain fat and fat has no ability to provide muscle function. By the time you are elderly SARCOPENIA prevents you from performing the most basic tasks of daily living, not to mention the risk of falls and other accidents.

If you don't start doing, you are going to start dying.

Obviously, the main way to prevent SARCOPENIA and live longer successfully is to exercise. You must find a way to use all your muscles. No one exercise will work for all, so do not despair. You do not have to become a body builder or a marathon runner.

○   Do you like to dance, walk, or ride a bike?

o   What did you like to do when you were a child? You will probably still like that or some version of it.

o   What sports do you like? Is it bowling, tennis, ping-pong, basketball, baseball, or golf?

o   Do you like group activities? If so, you would probably like yoga or Pilates.

o   If you are a quiet person and like your alone time, then get a small trampoline, hand weights and a big ball to bounce on.

Take the stairs and don't park right in front of the store. Walk! If you can walk three miles per hour at eighty, you have a ninety percent chance of living until you are ninety. If you can only walk one mile per hour at eighty, you have a ninety percent chance you will not see ninety.

Weight training and resistance training, not only builds bones and muscles, it gives you a forty percent less likely chance of heart attack, stroke, and sudden death.

I believe some form of resistance training is the best way to prevent SARCOPENIA.

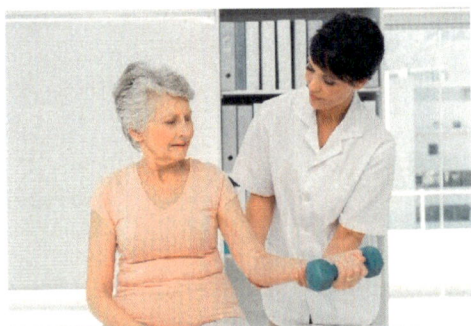

Resistance training is any exercise that causes the muscles to contract against an external resistance and with repetition muscles increase in strength, tone, mass, and endurance.

These are easy to add to your routines: arm raises, leg raises, squats, plank, push-ups, body rotation, and heel raises.

You don't have to do all of them every day. Work on your arms one day with dumbbells (or grab a can of beans from the pantry) for extra resistance. Work on your legs one day and the next try a few push-ups off the bathroom sink. Or get some exercise bands to work all areas of the body. Try resistant training vigorously just fifteen to thirty minutes a day!

Your body heals eight times faster when you exercise! **Just find something that MOVES you!** Here are a few more benefits of exercise:

- Controls weight
- Lowers blood pressure
- Improves quality of sleep
- Improves balance & coordination
- Improves flexibility
- Improves digestion
- Reduces osteoporosis
- Reduces joint stress & back pain
- Improves existing heart damage
- Decreases inflammation
- Improves immune function
- Improves liver health
- Improves insulin sensitivity (Type 2)
- Increases energy
- Reduces depression, anxiety, and stress
- Improves cognitive function

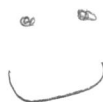

Because hormonal factors can significantly affect muscle mass, all adults over fifty should undergo annual blood testing to track their hormone levels. Look for supplements and natural solutions or alternatives.

Creatine, vitamin D, and plant protein have shown great promise in combating SARCOPENIA. Before taking protein supplements, get tested for Urea Cycle Disorder that reveals your ability to digest protein properly. Other nutrients such as omega-3 fatty acids and the amino acid glutamine have shown to improve a healthy muscle mass.

Inadequate intake of calories or protein can cause SARCOPENIA. Protein is very important, but as we age, digesting protein can be problematic. Combining protein with vegetables and fruits is easier on the digestive system than combining protein with starches. Limit refined carbs, cereals and most grains.

Your face can suffer as well. If you lose muscles, your skin hangs and sags and this can happen in the face as well. That is why many salons have the Non-Surgical Facelift Machine that retrains facial muscles providing a lifting appearance to the face. This is a type of EMS (electronic muscle stimulation) that was created for the face and it really helps you look younger.

SARCOPENIA is usually an 'old-persons' disease, but it doesn't have to be your future. A study from Brigham Young University reported that women who ran for 30 minutes five times a week, or biked regularly for 60 minutes, or strength trained for seventy-five minutes regularly reduced cellular aging by nine years.

The telomeres, the protective caps at the end of chromosomes that prevent age-acceleration, are damaged by inflammation. Exercise reduces inflammation which shortens telomeres. For more inflammation help, adopt the anti-inflammatory diet outlined in the chapter on SMOLDERING KILLER.

Stay active all the days of your life and you will not develop this debilitating, aging problem.

Eat healthy and find something that moves you and live a longer, younger life!

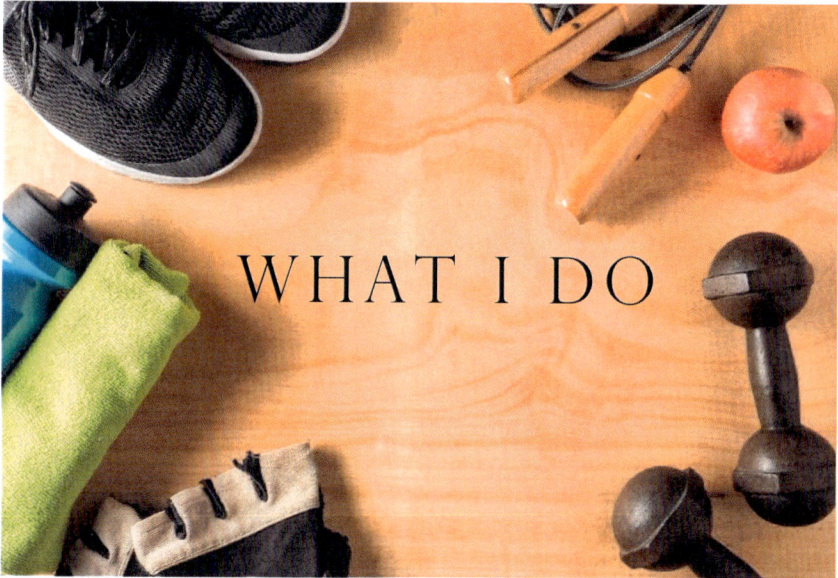

WHAT I DO

1. When on vacation, I will use the elliptical to run for fifteen to thirty minutes every other day, swim, and play golf.

2. Marathon exercising for hours causes a lot of free radical damage. This is cellular suicide. Working out in smaller quantities or shorter, but vigorous versions gives your body a chance to squelch these offenders before too much damage is done.

3. At home, I exercise on my bed and do leg lifts, bicycle, scissors, crunches, and sit ups.

4. I recently acquired a Full Body Vibration Machine. It promotes circulation, assists in weight loss, and increases bone density.

5. I use hand weights and resistance bands for my arms and upper body.

6. I had polio when I was five years old, and had to make annual visits to check the status for many years. They told me that I would have to exercise the rest of my life. I have!

7. I drink plant protein drinks with almond milk or collagen smoothies (with blueberries, juice of one lemon, greens, almond milk and half an avocado or MCT oil) for breakfast or a meal replacement.

8. I take, L-glutathione, pregnenolone, and omega-3 supplements.

9. I use an all-natural progesterone cream.

Chapter 4

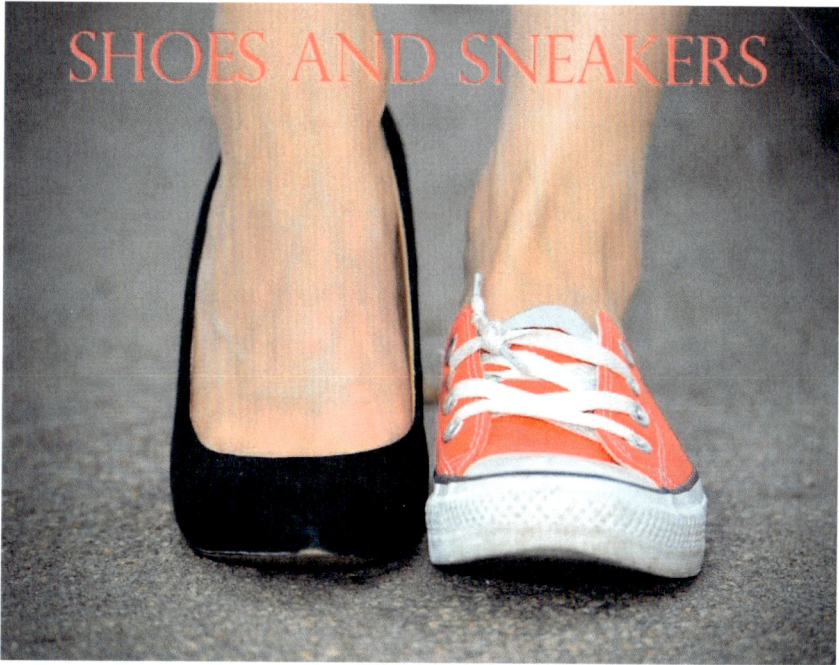

SHOES AND SNEAKERS

Did you know that your SHOES AND SNEAKERS are aging you and making you sick? **This chapter is going to be shocking, so don't skip this one.**

First, I will focus on the obvious negative effects that certain SHOES have on your health and well-being. Girl, I know you have those 'two-hour' SHOES in your closet. You just couldn't resist those beautiful booties even though they hurt your feet. Resist though, you must, if you want to live younger longer. SHOES that are too small or do not fit properly can cause a myriad of health problems. Here are just a few: corns, blisters, ingrown toenails, fallen arches, back pain, knee pain, arthritis, and bunions.

For someone my age, I actually have good-looking feet: no bunions, corns, or crooked toes. I think I owe this in part to my mother (she had beautiful feet with no issues), but mostly it was due to something I did at thirty-five. At that ripe old age, I thought I was over-the-hill. I was also pregnant, which may have contributed to my crazy thoughts.

I decided that I had better get rid of all my high heels before I injure myself or the baby. Remember, this was thirty-five years ago, and women were not routinely having children at that age like they are now. From then on, I focused on buying lower heels and comfort overlooking 'to-the-nines' on my feet.

No, I am not saying you have to wear granny SHOES! You do, however, need to be aware of how SHOES are affecting your health and longevity. Many manufacturers have stepped up to the plate and offer comfort without sacrificing fashion now. Obviously, sky-high heels are not good options for your back or hips. Even flat flats can affect your Achilles which can ultimately affect your arch.

It is best to have a variety of comfortable heel heights and toe fronts. Switch them out daily. The toe area should have room to wiggle your toes a little. **Who knows how much damage has been done by those pointy-toed-stilettos that Christian Dior introduced in the 1950s?** Remember, SHOES that are hurting your feet, are hurting your health.

Proper fitting SHOES AND SNEAKERS are an obvious healthy choice, but here's more helpful revelations you need to know. Have you heard of a mud room? They seem to be more common in the north where those pristine white snowfalls eventually turn into a frosty brown slush. The mud room is a place to remove your SHOES and hang your coats when coming in from the outside. Turns out, this is a genius addition to any home. Let me explain.

The University of Arizona did a study testing the inside and outside of SHOES AND SNEAKERS. **After only two weeks of wear, they found bacteria exceeding four hundred forty million units**. These bacteria also transferred onto tiles and other flooring in the home. According to their findings "bacteria thrive better on SHOES than toilets." Imagine these critters crawling around on your flooring:

- E. coli (causes intestinal and urinary tract infections)
- Meningitis
- Diarrhea
- Klebsiella pneumoniae
- Serratia ficaria (causes respiratory infections)
- C. difficile (causes colon infections)

Many cultures require you to leave your SHOES on the porch or in the entry way. They didn't need a study to tell them to do that. Now, though, there is proof (if you needed it) that walking outside in public areas where thousands of soles have been is hazardous to your health. Did you know that public bathrooms contain around two million bacteria per square inch?

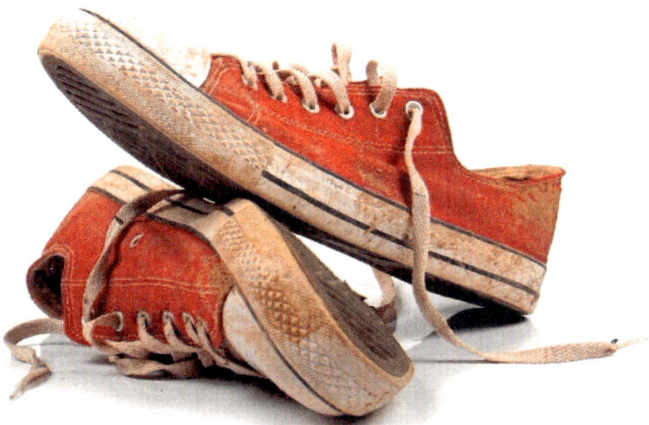

Dr. Rebecca Pruthi, DPM and Foot Health Expert, recommends five ways to combat shoe germs: 1) Remove your SHOES at the door to help detox your home. 2) Disinfect floors and shampoo rugs regularly. 3) Kick off SNEAKERS and throw them in the washing machine often. 4) Let SHOES air out rather than keeping them in a gym bag. 5) Store SHOES in a bag when placing them in your suitcase after cleaning them inside and out with disinfectant wipes.

Now, on to how SNEAKERS are damaging your health. Let's take a trip down memory lane to the 1870's. Imagine the lush green lawns and signature white costumes of croquet teams in England vying for the coveted winners' cup. Charles and I visited the Phyllis Court Club in Henley-on-Thames, England, recently where they still play croquet like they did over a hundred years ago.

It was like stepping back in time. It was lovely and relaxing. What does this have to do with SNEAKERS? Rubber-soled shoes were created for these clever athletes who wanted to ditch their leather shoes for something that would grip the ceramic croquet ball better. A better grip on their ball would allow them to smash their opponents' ball farther out of play!

Little did Charles Goodyear know that he was damaging the health of these and future athletes for centuries to come when he invented vulcanization? This process allowed him to mold rubber to a variety of materials like cloth. The U.K. croquet players were smitten and ditched their leather SHOES. Soon other athletes wanted some of these rubber wonders.

They called them daps, sand shoes, gutties, and plimsolls. Plimsoll was the name that stuck in England because it is a nautical term that describes the point at which the boat would take on water.

The point where the rubber sole met the cloth is where the wearer would take on water as well.

By 1916, in America, the U.S. Rubber company branded their plimsolls with a new name, and thus Keds were born. In 1917, the first high-top, rubber-soled trainer was introduced for basketball players. They were made by a Massachusetts shoemaker named Converse. Today, athletic SHOES AND SNEAKERS are engineered to perfection helping you run longer, jump higher, and even lose weight. So how could they possibly be damaging your health and longevity?

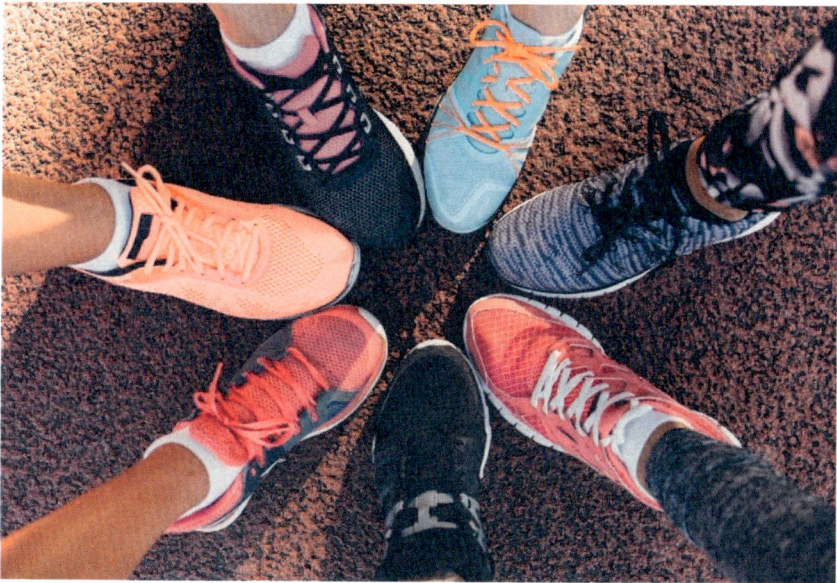

Here's the rest of the story, as Paul Harvey used to say. Look around and you will see a sea of rubber-soled SNEAKERS AND SHOES everywhere. They are worn to work, church, events, around the house, on planes, boats, and trains. They are no longer the coveted athletic shoe only. As we have left our leather shoe foundation, something caustic has happened.

Have you heard of grounding or earthing? New research is emerging that explains our need to get down to earth. Our ancestors used to be barefooted or use skins of animals for SHOES. Homes used to have dirt or stone floors. We used to walk to school, the market, or town square barefoot or in old-fashioned leather shoes. Literally, we used to touch the earth more. This connection with the earth actually causes a chemical reaction to take place in our bodies. Negatively charged electrons literally pass through our skin. Think of them as super anti-oxidants looking to squelch the destruction of free radicals.

You probably don't think about it, but, you are a bio-electrical being. Everything is electrical: your heart, your lungs, your brain, etc. Without this negative-charged energy, inflammation, thickened blood, mitochondrial dysfunction, and auto immune problems spread out of control. Free radicals, also known as ROS (reactive oxygen species), are positively charged, so connecting with the earth neutralizes these bad boys. If you are wearing SNEAKERS, the rubber does not conduct this energy, it actually shields you from it. They theorize this has contributed to the massive increase in bodily inflammation.

Basically, we live inside a giant battery (the earth and the surrounding atmosphere); the earth having the negative charge and the ionosphere sixty miles up having the positive charge. This battery is constantly being charged with electrons (energy) from lightning, sun radiation, and molten-core (center of earth) heat.

As a human living in this battery, your bodily functions are powered by these same electrons. Think of yourself as a little Energizer Bunny that needs recharging every day. Dr. Joseph Mercola says, "Just about every tissue in your body is energized with electrical currents, including your immune system, nervous system, brain, muscles, heart, lungs, and even your behavior."

According to James Oschman, PhD. of Biology, and his research published in *The Journal of Inflammation Research*, grounding has anti-aging benefits. The dominate **theory of aging** "emphasizes cumulative damage caused by ROS produced during normal metabolism or prolonged in response to pollutants, poisons, or injury. We hypothesize an anti-aging effect of grounding that is based on a living matrix reaching every part of the body and that is capable of delivering anti-oxidant electrons to sites where tissue integrity might be comprised by reactive oxidants from any source." Who knew going barefoot could slow down aging?

Other benefits of grounding are:

- Improved sleep
- Reduced pain
- Shifting autonomic nervous system from cortisol producing
- Normalizing the day-night cortisol rhythm
- Reduced stress
- Increased heart rate variability
- Reduced blood viscosity

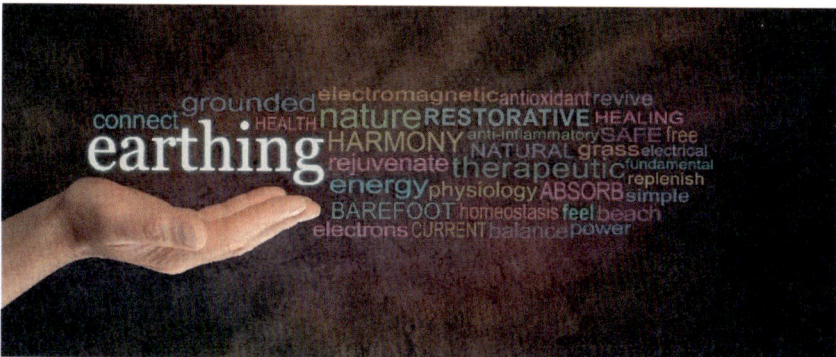

The Journal of Environmental and Public Health reports: "grounding or earthing the human body may be an essential element in the health equation along with sunshine, clean air and water, nutritious food, and physical activity." Please check out the legendary work Clint Ober has done and his YouTube video: *Grounded*. He and Dr. Stephen Sinatra (cardiologist specialist) also co-authored a ground-breaking book called *Earthing*.

So, take off those SHOES AND SNEAKERS! Here are the surfaces that ground you: 1) sand, preferably on the beach, 2) grass, preferably wet, 3) bare soil, 4) concrete or brick that has not been sealed, 5) ceramic tile.

Walk your dog or yourself barefooted. Take your next vacation on the beach. If you live near a beach, go barefoot walking on it more often. Just go barefoot in your back yard early in the morning when the dew is fresh. If you don't have a backyard, find a nearby park or green space that is pesticide-free. Don't be afraid of the dirt, walk in it.

Other options are buying special grounding SHOES or grounding pads that can be attached to the bottoms of your feet. Grounding mats are also available that can fit under your desk. Grounding sheets can help you get a really good night's rest. There are even grounding yoga mats. Buy real leather-soled SHOES to keep grounded.

Who knew SHOES AND SNEAKERS could be so damaging to your health?

If you want to live younger longer, take a new look at your love affair with SHOES AND SNEAKERS and make some much-needed changes!

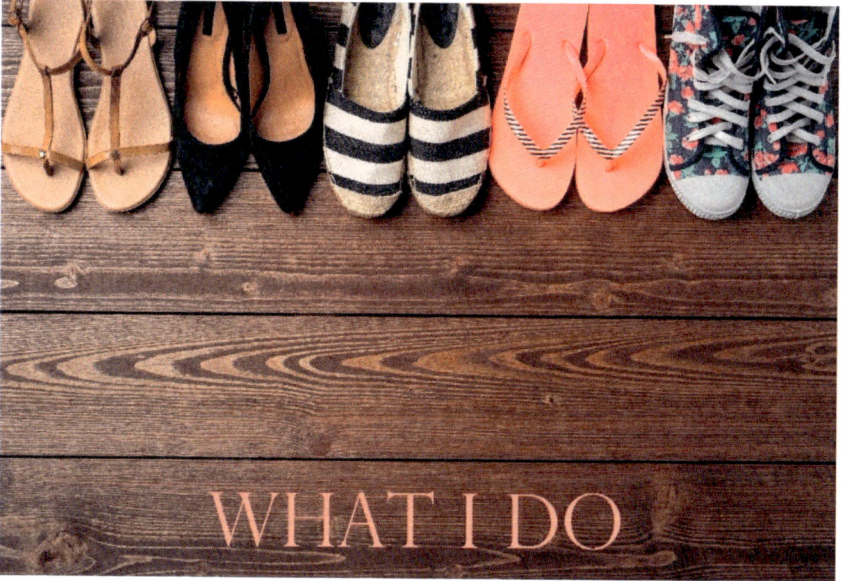

WHAT I DO

1. I am not a big fan of SNEAKERS, so I only wear them when going to the gym or playing golf.

2. I wear a variety of SHOES, boots, and sandals each week.

3. Most of our vacations are on a beach somewhere. We have also just discovered Sedona, AZ. Apparently, it has swirling centers of energy vortices where you can experience the same high level of energizing.

4. I keep wipes in my car to clean my shoes after going to malls and public bathrooms.

5. I love to work in the yard pulling weeds and gardening. Of course, I am barefooted because we don't use harmful pesticides.

6. We spend a lot of time in our outdoor living area with a floor of natural stone over concrete. No need for SHOES there.

7. I have a grounding yoga mat and we have grounding mats placed on the floor under our desks.

8. I love to take walks barefooted in the rain.

9. I roll in the grass with Merlot. It's not what you think. Merlot is my dog. Sometimes we just go out in the backyard, sit on the grass and get some sun. Occasionally, he will roll around in the grass, so I join him for a little earthing. ☺

10. Our home has a mudroom. We leave our shoes there or clean them with wipes. All our shoe polish and leather creams are kept there as well.

11. I have a shoe cabinet with doors, where all my boots and shoes are stored.

12. When traveling, Charles and I place our SHOES in bags or I just put all mine in a large purse to carry on the plane.

Chapter 5

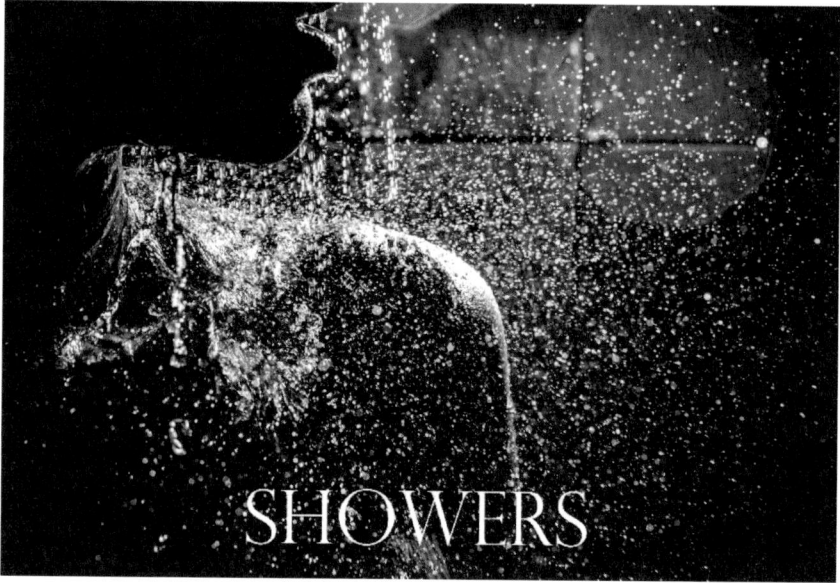

SHOWERS

Yes, that hot, steamy shower you take each day may be making you sick! Have you heard of the *Microbiome Project*? **It's a study about what critters are living in your showerhead.** By critters I mean bacteria and mold. The Fierer Laboratory at the University of Colorado in Boulder is trying to determine if the microbial life is really detrimental to your health. Apparently, nontuberculous mycobacterial (NTM), which is found naturally in soil, has found its way to showerheads. While most of the one hundred seventy species of NTM are harmless, some cause severe lung infections in those with weakened immune systems. Legionella pneumophila causes a type of pneumonia called Legionnaire's disease. This bacterium has also found its way into showerheads.

Atypical mycobacteria are all around us in the soil and water and continued exposure to these tiny aliens actually builds our immune system. The problem comes, though, when we are constantly over exposed from a contaminated showerhead. The daily barrage of air borne droplets of water small enough to enter our lungs could be too much to overcome for some.

Do you put your head under the showerhead to let the steaming hot water cascade through your hair and over your face? Does that water get into your eyes and mouth? Did you breathe while doing this? If you have a compromised immune system, this is probably not a good idea. If you have any open wounds, this is probably not a good idea. If you are wearing contacts, this is probably not a good idea. Infections of the skin, lungs, eyes, sinuses, lymph nodes, etc. can come from exposure to atypical mycobacteria. Take a bath instead, SHOWERS could be making you sick.

According to *National Jewish Health*, thirty thousand NTM infections are diagnosed each year and the cure rate is only fifty percent. Unlike TB, it is spread through the environment, not from person to person. They recommend that you clean your showerhead by soaking it in vinegar and water and even replace it periodically. They also recommend that if you have lung problems, to wear a mask when gardening.

Scientists at Manchester University in the U.K. studied the bathroom scum in SHOWERS and found the bacteria and fungi were linked to a range of illnesses. Dr. Paul McDermott, a former Safety Executive, summarized some of the findings for the *Mirror*:

- Eyes: "Dirty shower water in the eyes can lead to an infection called Keratitis or inflammation of the cornea which is linked to Malassezia fungi." Another bacterium called acanthamoeba "can cause this painful eye infection that can lead to blindness." The treatments could last for years and even involve corneal graft in severe cases. Contact wearers are more susceptible because of the minor scratches on the cornea. Also, "the acanthamoeba is attracted to the contact lenses and any natural bacteria living on the lenses can serve as a food source, enabling them to survive." Do not wear contact lenses when taking SHOWERS!

- Ears: Another bug discovered is the Pseudomonas aeruginosa bacterium which leads to 'swimmers ear.' This bacterium strikes usually when someone is sick or rundown. "For healthy people who may pick up an infection from a shower or swimming pool, they can generally get over it, but for certain patients receiving treatment in hospitals, infections can be much more serious, and even life threatening."

- Lungs: Legionella bacteria thrive in the warm waters of the shower and are inhaled into the lungs. The flu-like symptoms are often misdiagnosed, and if not treated quickly, can be fatal. Those with respiratory issues, compromised immune systems, and the elderly are at high risk. "There is a very simple test that can give a diagnosis within an hour. The key is that people do ask for that test if they are genuinely concerned that they have the disease."

- Hair: If you've never cleaned or replaced your showerhead, it could be giving you dandruff. The study identified fungi called Malassezia restricta that lives in the black gunge in the shower head. These organisms have been linked to skin infections and dandruff. Folliculitis is another nasty problem caused from the water squirting out of the shower. Visible spots, rashes, and patches of itchy skin around hair follicles plague many people now.

- Stomach – Digestive System: A study done at Lancaster University reported that one in ten showerheads were contaminated with mycobacterium avium subspecies paratububerculosis. To make a long story short, this bacterium has been linked to Chrohn's disease which affects the digestive system. Running the shower for a short period may help reduce contamination.

- Blood: Another germ is found in the biofilm that collects on showerheads and in baths called Pseudomonas aeruginosa. "Pseudomonas are opportunist pathogens and those most at risk of infection are people who aren't well and those whose immune systems sadly don't have the ability to fight it." It is resistant to many antibiotics which make it difficult to treat and cure. This bug is common in hospitals and deaths generally occur when it leads to septicemia.

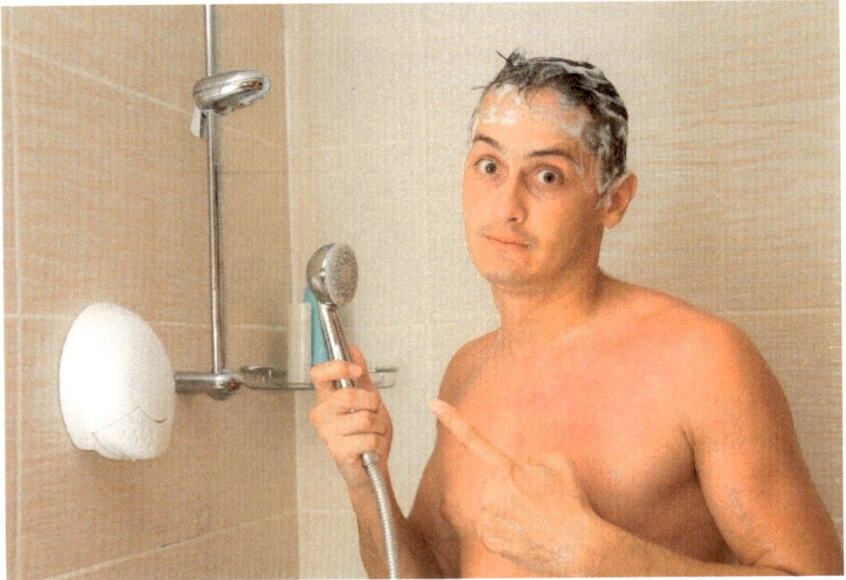

What about your skin? Health experts are now recommending that you should avoid showers after beauty treatments like microdermabrasion, surgery, peels, or CO_2 laser treatments. The concern is that under these circumstances, germs may have an easier way in.

New research from Saint Antonio Abate Hospital in Naples, Italy, found that contaminated shower water can cause skin irritations after operations or beauty treatments. Use filtered, sterile water for cleansing the face or body until the treated area is healed completely to avoid infection.

Mildew, mold, fungi, soap scum, bacteria, pink stuff, biofilm, etc. are lurking in your shower like a hungry mountain lion in a tree waiting to pounce on his prey. OK, maybe that is a little dramatic. I'm just trying to get your attention and make you aware of this potentially dangerous situation. Your immune system could be compromised from STRESS, SLEEPLESSNESS, SUGAR, SICKNESS, or whatever, which could make you prone to infection from SHOWERS.

Epsom or Himalayan salt baths are healthy alternatives to SHOWERS and can even help you recover and reboot. An Epsom Salt sitz bath should actually be part of a regular regimen to stay healthy in any case. Epsom Salt is rich in magnesium sulfate and magnesium is the second-most abundant element in your cells. Most Americans have a magnesium deficiency due to poor diet habits which leads to a calcium to magnesium imbalance. For optimum health it should be two to one (calcium to magnesium), but for most Americans it is five to one.

The National Academy of Sciences says that magnesium deficiency leads to heart disease, stroke, osteoporosis, arthritis, digestive issues, stress-related illnesses, and chronic fatigue. While sitz baths are known to help alleviate pain, heal skin problems, reduce infection and soothe hemorrhoids, you will also receive this beneficial mineral as it penetrates the skin into your body. Clean your tub with vinegar and water, fill to six inches with hot water, and add two cups of salts and your favorite essential oils.

Consider taking more baths with essential oils. Adding them to bath salts helps them disperse more evenly.

- Frankincense helps improve cell regeneration, treats dry skin, and reverses the signs of aging.
- Tangerine is a great remedy for acne and skin impurities.
- Lavender, geranium, and myrrh are also good for skin rejuvenation.
- Bergamot soothes skin irritations, kills germs and bacteria, and relieves joint and muscle pain.
- Evening Primrose reduces inflammation and improves eczema, psoriasis and atopic dermatitis.
- Ylang Ylang oil is great for a relaxing bath and those who have insomnia.
- Patchouli oil reduces the appearance of wrinkles, blemishes, or problem skin areas, as well as, calms emotions.

For you shower lovers, remove your showerhead and soak it in vinegar and water for two hours. While it is soaking, spray your shower with a blend of vinegar and water. Replace your showerhead yearly. There are also showerhead filters available that help solve the contamination issues.

Who knew that taking SHOWERS could be so dangerous to your health and longevity?

If you want to live younger longer keep those SHOWERS and showerheads clean and take more baths!!

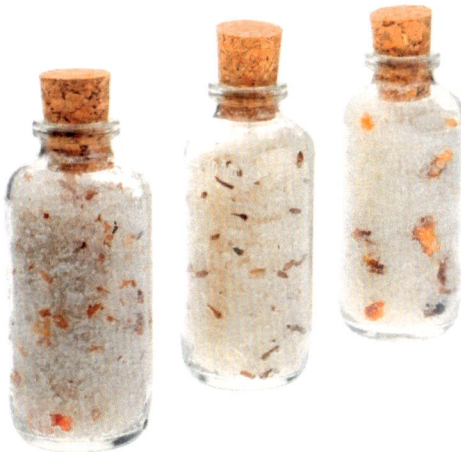

WHAT I DO

1. I prefer taking baths. I have my essential oils right next to the tub for easy access.

2. My salts are sitting in pretty containers along with candles on the tub surround.

3. I buy dried herbs like lavender, chamomile, and geranium to mix with my Epsom salts.

4. I save dried flower petals (especially rose petals) to mix with Himalayan salts.

5. I don't wear my contacts when taking a shower.

6. I like to add essential oils to coconut oil for moisturizing my legs and arms after a bath or shower.

7. We have a showerhead filter, but still change our showerheads every couple of years.

8. I use vinegar and water to pre-clean the shower to kill off mold and bacteria.

Chapter 6

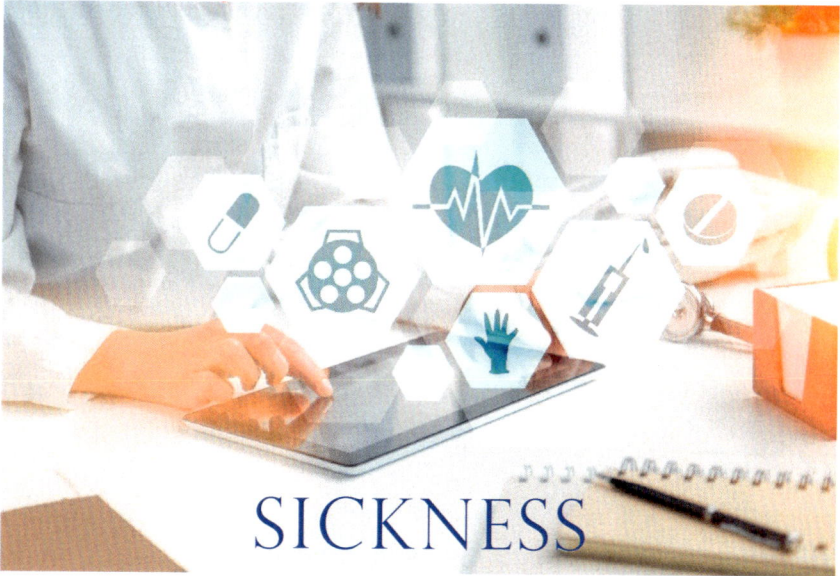

SICKNESS

The Center for Disease and Prevention (CDC) reports that as of 2012 about half of the adults in America (117,000,000) had one or more chronic health conditions. Astonishingly, one in four adults had two or more chronic health conditions. Two chronic conditions, cancer and heart disease, account for almost all deaths.

The CDC also reports that arthritis is the most common cause of disability and fifty-four million people have been diagnosed with this crippling SICKNESS. Diabetes is the leading cause of kidney failure, lower-limb amputation, and blindness among adults.

It doesn't take a rocket scientist to know that SICKNESS or disease or illnesses will age you.

You probably know someone who has had a heart attack, stroke, or cancer and the toll it has taken on their life. So why do you want to get SICK? What? You say you don't want to get SICK, yet you are 1) **overweight**, 2) **physically inactive**, 3) **eat poorly**, and some of you even 4) **smoke**. Scientists and physicians have known that these four lifestyle answers determine your chance of illness and chronic disease since the *Potsdam Study* was completed over twenty years ago.

You will find disturbing information on being overweight in SIZE MATTERS, why you are eating poorly in STARVATION, what happens when you are not active in SARCOPENIA, and the scoop on SMOKING in this book. If you follow even some of my advice and make changes, you will see improvement in your health and longevity. SICKNESS does not have to be your FUTURE. This chapter will focus on improving your immune system for even better results.

Hippocrates said, "All disease begins in the GUT."

- A word about GUT HEALTH: By now you may have heard the highway to health is through your gut. Eighty percent of your immune system is in your gut and gut bacteria are your first line of defense. There are around 100 trillion bacteria in your body and ten times more bacterial cells than human cells.
- This microbiome is a universe of organisms that communicate with the immune system. For the sake of time, I will just say there are good bacteria that improve digestion and send nutrients to cells and bad bacteria that cause inflammation and disease.

The BAD BACTERIA love to eat SUGAR and STARCHES. And if you feed them a lot, they can even send messages to your brain to activate cravings for even more. So, you could say the bad microbiomes in my gut made me eat that donut! ☺

When you start feeding the good microbiomes with fruits and vegetables, they will eventually gain control of your cravings.

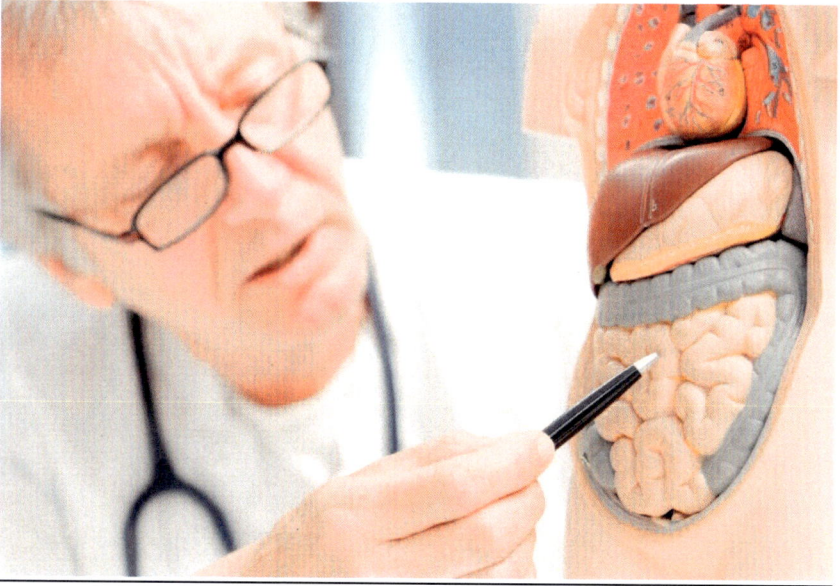

The GOOD BACTERIA love PROBIOTICS! Probiotics are foods or supplements that contain live strains of microbes that target a particular health benefit. They aid in digestion, assist immune function, control inflammation, prevent cancer, regulate lipids and metabolism, relieve allergies, improve skin conditions, improve nutrient utilization, and prevent hypertension.

These foods include: YOGURT, KEFIR, MISO, NATTO, TEMPEH, SAUERKRAUT, KIMCHEE, FERMENTED VEGIES, ROOT & GINGER BEERS, OLIVES, PULKE, KOMBUCHA, BUTTERMILK, RAW WHEY, RAW VINEGARS, SOURDOUGH, ESSENE BREAD, BEER, AND WINE.

The GOOD BACTERIA love PREBIOTICS! Prebiotics are foods that are not digested by human enzymes but are fermented by intestinal micro-flora stimulating the growth and activity of intestinal bacteria.

These foods include: JERUSALEM ARTICHOKES, CHICORY, GARLIC, BANANAS, FRUIT, SOYBEANS, BURDOCK ROOT, SUGAR MAPLE, CHIVES, PEAS, LEGUMES, EGGPLANT, HONEY, GREEN TEA, YOGURT, COTTAGE CHEESE, AND KEFIR.

A word about YOGURT: In the 'old days' my grandparents drank buttermilk but no one had heard of yogurt. Now, everyone has heard of this healthy food, but leave it to the U.S. food industry to mess it up.

They've added sugar, fruit, and flavorings that destroy all its benefits because they kill off the good bacteria. Add plain, unflavored yogurt to your shopping list if you want to make your gut happy. For those with a sweet tooth, make a dessert by sweetening with honey or stevia and topping with fruit and nuts.

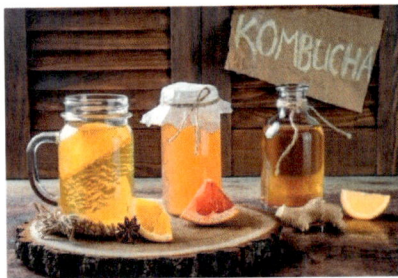

A word about KOMBUCHA: Kombucha is fast becoming the new 'soda' of the health food industry. It originated over two thousand years ago in China and they refer to it as the "Imperial Health Elixir." It is a fermented sparkling beverage made of black tea (it can also be made of green tea) sweetened with cane sugar, fruit sugar, or honey.

The fermentation produces probiotics, B vitamins, vinegar, and enzymes. The good bacteria in Kombucha produce cellulose which acts like a "shield to cells" according to Dr. Axe an expert on gut health. This wonder drink produces anti-oxidants that fight inflammation and disease.

It improves digestion, lung health, and mental well-being. It also alleviates diabetic symptoms and lowers tri-glycerides and cholesterol. Try the 'in' soda, Kombucha, and improve your immune system.

If the highway to your health is indeed through the gut, America is in serious trouble! The Standard American Diet is truly SAD! SEVENTY-FIVE PERCENT of it consists of refined carbohydrates which have no benefit to the microbiome in the lower gut.

There are ten times more of them than of you. Why not partner with these little fellows so you can avoid SICKNESS by improving your immune system and enjoy a long and healthy life?

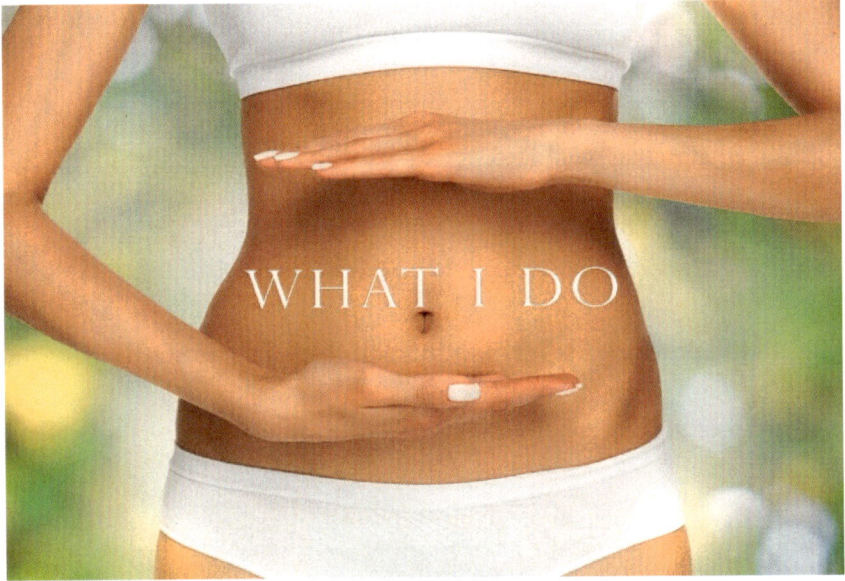

WHAT I DO

1. I eat fermented veggies and sauerkraut.

2. I cook with buttermilk and make sauces and dips with yogurt.

3. I drink green tea and red wine.

4. I love artichokes, peas, eggplant, and legumes.

5. I love honey and gluten-free toast with hot green tea for a snack.

6. I do not eat cake, donuts, cupcakes, or cookies made with sugar and flour.

7. I love the new probiotic drinks trending in the health-food aisles and stores.

8. I drink raw apple cider vinegar (1 tbsp.) with water in the morning.

9. I eat mostly a Paleo diet.

10. I take VSL#3 Probiotic Medical Food and Garden of Life probiotics.

Chapter 7

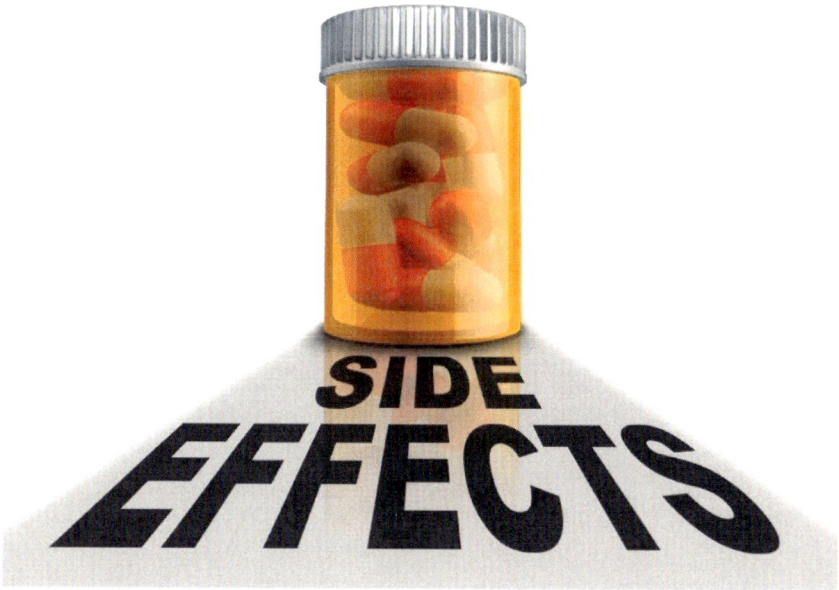

Every year four and a half million Americans visit the doctor's office or emergency room because of adverse prescription drug SIDE EFFECTS. Another two million patients already hospitalized, suffer ill effects of prescription drugs annually. **Every year, SIDE EFFECTS cause <u>one hundred thousand</u> deaths making prescription drugs the fourth leading cause of deaths in the U.S. Illegal drugs only kill ten thousand people annually.**

Even though prescription drugs undergo stringent testing, a number of SIDE EFFECTS are allowed. These SIDE EFFECTS affect each person differently because of many variables like: height, weight, age, gender, ethnicity, and overall health. After testing by the Food and Drug Administration (FDA), if the drug has more advantages than disadvantages, the drug is approved.

You've seen the commercials on TV and some of them scare the bejeebies out of me. They speak of bleeding, nerve pain, digestive issues, death, cancer, heart attacks, disabilities, nausea, fainting, thoughts of suicide, liver damage, kidney damage, etc. as though they were common or natural and to be expected. **You don't have a prescription drug deficiency.** For instance, food and exercise are better choices to increase bone density than a laboratory concocted drug with SIDE EFFECTS.

I'm not going to be preachy here, but I think you can see that the SIDE EFFECTS of prescription drugs can be aging you. So, why not be proactive and start living a healthier, holistic life while you can? Don't look into the future and believe that prescription drugs are the ultimate answer for your health problems as you age. "Rubbish," as my husband would say! There is enough information out there that proves your body can heal itself or remain healthy as you age when given the right ingredients. This is not to say that you should never go to the doctor or take a prescription drug.

A word about antibiotic resistance: The World Health Organization (WHO) says that antibiotic resistance is one of the biggest threats to global health, food security, and development

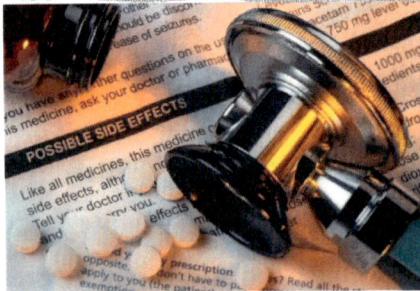

today. The WHO explains that antibiotic resistance occurs when bacteria change in response to the use of these medicines. Bacteria become antibiotic resistant, not humans or animals.

Pneumonia, tuberculosis, blood poisoning, and gonorrhea are becoming harder or sometimes impossible to treat. Misuse and overuse of antibiotics and poor prevention practices lead to antibiotic resistance.

If you have turned to antibiotics every time you were ill, by the time you are of boomer age, these once life-saving drugs may not work. **The Centers for Disease Control and Prevention report that at least 23,000 people die each year due to antibiotic resistance.**

By now you have heard that the use of antibiotics affects your gut biome which is the seat of your immune system because they destroy the good bacteria, as well as, the bad bacteria. If impairing your immune system is not frightening enough, more studies are being done on the effects of antibiotics on brain health. A study by Max-Delbrück-Centre for *Molecular Medicine* in Germany revealed a slowdown in brain cell development in the hippocampus which is responsible for memory and controlling the nervous system.

Antibiotic resistance, destruction of your immune system, and brain cell impairment won't necessarily be a warning from your doctor or listed on an information guide. You must take charge of your health and stay informed. This is an important example of the negative SIDE EFFECTS you will encounter. It has become a world-wide health issue so I thought it important to touch base on it.

You must be aware of everything that has to do with your body, your health, and aging. Be sure to read the *Medication Guide* that comes with your prescription as it will alert you to most of the SIDE EFFECTS. Research your health problem to learn alternative, natural options for improvement.

Be alert, stay aware, and try to avoid the snare of prescription drug SIDE EFFECTS when possible.

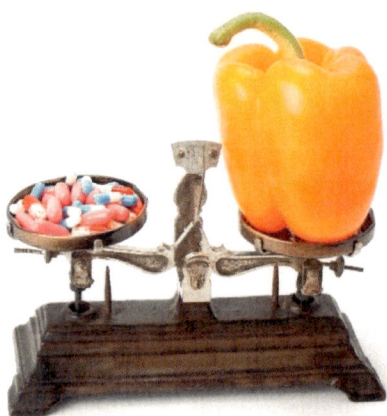

WHAT I DO

1. I read all labels.

2. I stay informed by reading articles and newsletters.

3. I am so in tune with my body, that I know when I'm not feeling well so I rest, drink green tea, broth, and juice and do whatever else may remedy the problem.

4. I rarely get sick, but did go to Mexico recently and got a bladder infection. And yes, I had to take antibiotics to get rid of it. Also, I took extra probiotics for the urinary tract.

5. I eat organic at home, take vitamins and probiotics, juice, and make smoothies every day. Seventy-five percent of my food intake is fruits and vegetables. I eat plenty of good fats like avocado (everyday), butter, olive oil, and coconut oil. All this gives my body the ingredients it needs to heal and prevent disease.

6. I avoid sugar and starches (white stuff).

Chapter 8

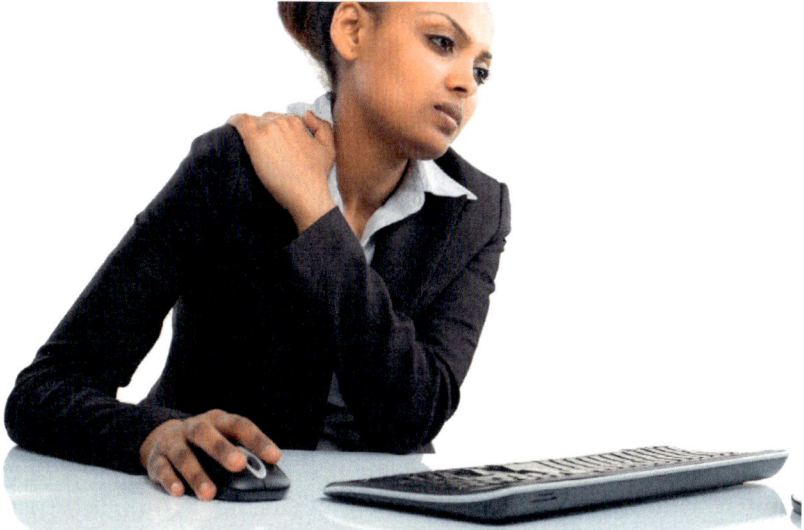

SITTING

SITTING is the new SMOKING. Perhaps you've heard that alarming phrase lately? Let me explain where it came from. Do you work in an office? Then, you probably sit (between drive time and office time) anywhere from thirteen to fifteen hours a day. If you are my age, you may remember when SMOKING was thought to be healthy and everyone smoked. We now know that is not true.

When SITTING was first presented as a health risk by Dr. James Levine to his Mayo Clinic colleagues, they rebuked his findings as well. Since then, over ten thousand studies have surfaced that have shown him to be correct. **Shockingly, reports show that for every hour you sit down, your life expectancy decreases by two hours.** In comparison, for every cigarette you smoke, your life expectancy only decreases eleven minutes.

For more details, get his book: *Get Up! Why Your Chair Is Killing You and What You Can Do About It.*

You may think that if you go to the gym a few times a week or run every day, you are OK. Well, think again. Apparently, it's the continuous hours of the seated position and bodily inactivity that is the problem. **When the body is crammed into a chair, cellular mechanisms that push fuel into your cells get turned off.**

According to Dr. Levine, when you stand, within 90 seconds the muscular and cellular systems that process blood sugar, triglycerides, and cholesterol (which are mediated by insulin) are activated. You and I know that SITTING is bad for the back, but Dr. Levine says it damages your wrist, arms, and your metabolism and causes toxic build up as well. Who knew that SITTING was more hazardous to your health than SMOKING?

SITTING was not meant to be a way of life. The human body was meant to be active and moving all day long. If you examine the lives of the centurions in the 'Blue Zones,' they walk everywhere, grow and/or raise their own food, and are highly social. I don't think any of them work in an office and sit at a desk all day long. Dr. Levine recommends that you sit no longer than fifty minutes at a time. Standing up and moving around for ten minutes each hour is the bare minimum you should do.

Who knew that being an office worker was more dangerous than working construction? Fortunately, the workplace is changing by offering standing stations and stand-up desks. There are bracelets that encourage you to take ten thousand steps a day. I've even heard there are meetings now where no one sits, they just move around and conduct business.

That is music to the ears of the author of *Deskbound: Standing Up to a Sitting World.* Dr. Kelly Starrett, a Ph.D. in physical therapy, explains that just standing up is not sufficient.

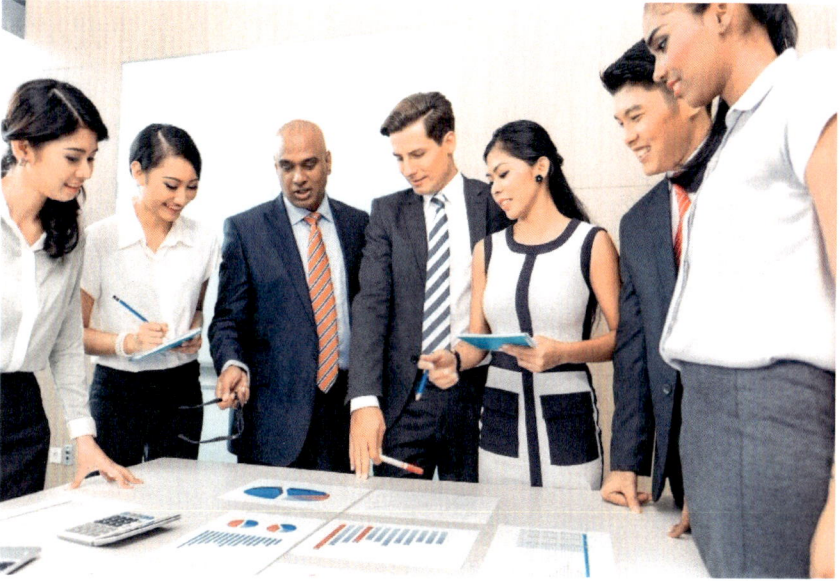

Your body was created for a full range of motion to optimize your physiology. In his book, he helps you create a movement-rich environment around the workplace. SITTING tall is SITTING properly which is like looking over a fence. A great office exercise is squeezing your buttocks. He also suggests sitting on the floor cross-legged and working or sitting on a ball instead of a chair.

Another researcher from NASA, Dr. Joan Vernikos, wrote another compelling book: *Sitting Kills, Moving Heals*. She explains the science behind the fact that even if you work out five times a week for thirty minutes each time, you will not have optimal health if you sit most of the time.

The secret to her research was the fact that frequent intermittent interactions with gravity that interrupts your SITTING was the key to health and vitality.

Apparently, one week in space is equal to one year of aging on earth, which amounts to a ten-fold acceleration of aging in a gravity-free environment.

She said that what became abundantly clear to her very quickly was that gravity plays a big role in our physiological function and the aging process.

She goes on to say that we were designed to squat and to kneel and sitting is ok but not continuously. Think of SITTING in your chair as being in outer space or "quasi-microgravity." It's not how many hours you sit; it's how many times you get up. She suggests at least thirty-two times a day or every twenty minutes!

All that to say this: SITTING and the lack of movement is aging you and probably making you fat. Yes, I said the non-politically correct word: fat. Did you know the mere act of standing up activates the enzyme, lipoprotein lipase, which rushes out to attach to fat in your bloodstream and takes it to muscles to be used as energy? Just standing activates fat burning. Wow!

You may not work in an office, but you sit on the couch or your favorite chair all day. You may even be crocheting or sewing, but you are still SITTING.

You may even say that you are not feeling good or you have pulled a muscle or have muscle cramps. Hello, it's because you are not standing up and moving. It's time to get up and get off your bum if you want to live a younger, longer life. Check out my chapter on SARCOPENIA for great ways to add movement back into your life.

Stop SITTING so much and live a younger, longer, slimmer life!

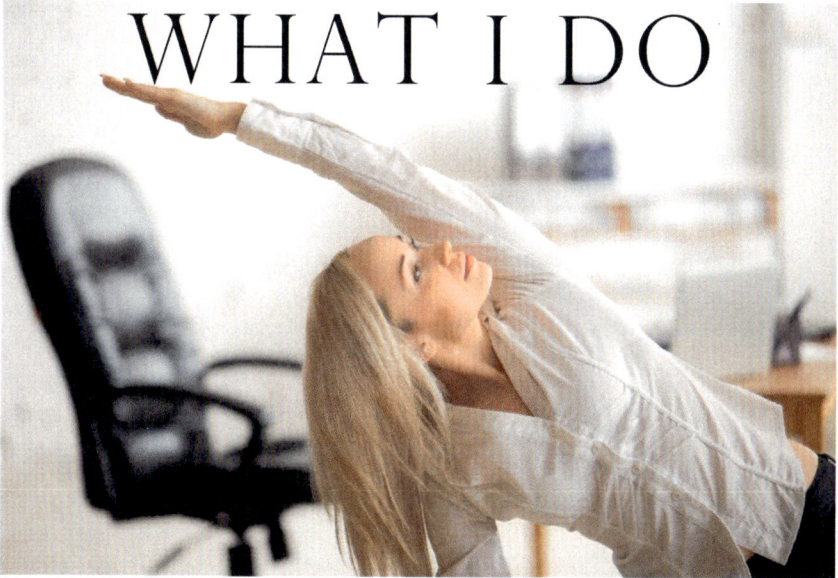

WHAT I DO

1. I have Full Body Vibration Machine that I try to use every day. It was developed with NASA technology to improve bone density and muscle atrophy for astronauts after space travel. It is classified as a Class 1 medical device and found to improve circulation, mental awareness, flexibility, range of motion, toning firming, weight management, stress relief, and pain relief in joints and muscles. I think this is one of the best investments for senior health, but would also help those that find themselves SITTING all day.

2. I stand on matts most all day long with my job, so SITTING only becomes a problem when I am writing. I get bored easily and get up often.

3. I try to stretch every day with fluid movements much like tai chi. I can still touch my toes!

4. I exercise at home with hand weights and resistance bands.

5. I love to dance around the house.

Chapter 9

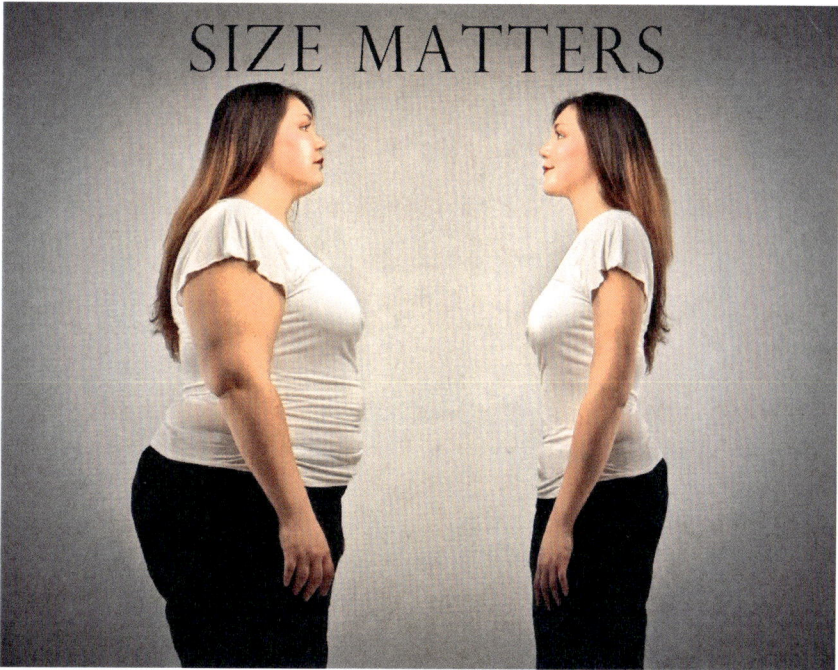

By now you should know your SIZE MATTERS. **Obesity is the leading cause of death in the U.S. and for that matter, the world!** But wait, there's more. The Center for Disease Control and Prevention reports, "people who have obesity, compared to those with normal or healthy weight, are at increased risk for many serious diseases and health conditions including the following:"

- High blood pressure (hypertension)
- High LDL cholesterol, low HDL (good cholesterol), high triglycerides
- Type 2 diabetes
- Coronary heart disease

- Stroke

- Gall bladder disease and kidney problems

- Osteoarthritis (bone-in-joint degeneration)

- Sleep apnea and breathing problems

- Low quality of life

- Mental illness (depression, anxiety, and other mental conditions)

- Body pain and difficulty with physical functioning

- Some cancers (endometrial, breast, colon, kidney, gallbladder, and liver)

A recent report in the *New England Journal of Medicine* emphasized that the U.S. leads the world in childhood and adult obesity. I'm sure this is no surprise to anyone. All you have to do is to look around the mall, restaurant, ballpark, football stadium, movie theater, or church and count the number of overweight people as compared to the normal weight people. **Columbia University reports that one in five deaths is due to obesity.** If you are overweight, obese, or morbidly obese, you know it. The question is: "What are you willing to do about it?"

Even though weight loss is a sixty-five-billion-dollar business in the U.S., people are getting fatter and fatter. Yes, I said fatter! I don't want to sugar-coat this because it's so serious. ☺ As Americans leave the kitchen to pass through the drive-thru because it is cheaper and easier than cooking at home, they consume more energy-dense food than they can burn off. As comfort food becomes more important than healthy food, even more energy is consumed that cannot be expended. Finally, as activities now are based around food engagement instead of physical engagement, even more energy is stored. Stored energy is fat, fuel for future use, but for most, it never gets used. One of my professors said that food is the fuel that will determine your future. What does your future look like?

If you are overweight, obese, or extreme obese your future is in the list of diseases I listed earlier. According to the National Institute on Health, two-thirds of adults in America are overweight or obese. More than one in three adults are obese and one in twenty adults are considered extreme obese. Unfortunately, even one-third of adolescents are overweight or obese. Extreme obesity (BMI over forty) has risen 350 percent in the past few years.

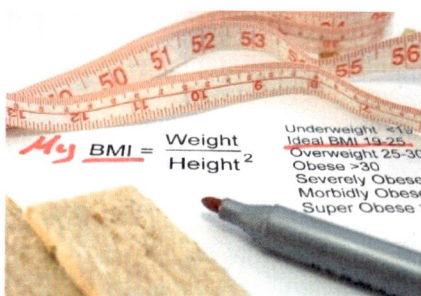

In order to slow down the aging process and live happier and healthier longer, you must achieve and maintain a normal BMI. BMI (body mass index) is the measurement of choice now. Insurance companies and physicians consider it a more accurate accounting since it includes your height, weight, gender, and even your ethnicity. In the UK, the government medical service now refuses certain surgeries if the patient is obese according to BMI. Hello America! This is coming here. It's time to take charge of your health and lose weight. You can find a BMI calculator online at *mayoclinic.org*.

This may give you a little incentive. Three frightening facts about FAT:

1. Dr. Daniel Amen, psychiatrist and brain health expert, explains that as your weight goes up, the size of your brain goes down. This causes less function in the frontal cortex, where you think. It affects your thoughts, planning, empathy, judgement, organization, impulse, learning from mistakes – basically everything that makes you human.

2. Fat stores toxins which produce cytokines in the blood which are inflammatory messengers that disrupt normal hormonal production. It is associated with causing depression, inducing cell death, and interrupting stress hormone production. Alzheimer's, Parkinson's, multiple sclerosis, and autism have elevated cytokine production. Obesity doubles the risk in men, and triples the risk in women to get Alzheimer's.

3. The more body fat you have, the less your ability to produce adiponectin. Adiponectin is a protein produced in fat cells that plays a pivotal role in energy metabolism, but the more fat you have the less you can make. In my words, the more body fat you have, the fatter you will become. You must lose body fat to increase your metabolism.

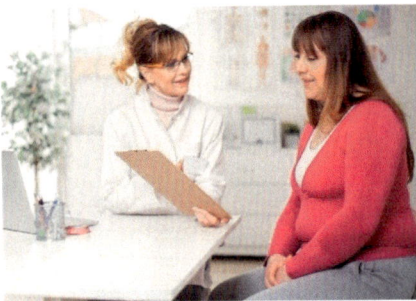

Throughout this book you will get loads of information on how to lose weight and get healthier, but here are a few more nuggets. Health coaches know that you just can't restrict calories and lose weight forever.

We know you can't even exercise your way out of a bad diet and lose weight. We promote a more holistic approach that includes the big picture of your whole life. Here are three of my approaches to losing weight that you can incorporate with the rest of the healthy tips to come:

- To lose weight permanently, you must examine 'the why' you are putting food into your mouth. Are you really hungry? Or are you mad, sad, trained to clean your plate, anxious, impulsive, compulsive, envious, self-hating, unforgiving, fitting-in, shameful, craving something or someone, stressed, lonely, or you fill in the blank? Emotional eating is the number one reason for obesity.

- For permanent weight loss, you must examine 'the what' you are eating and what it is doing to you or for you. Before you put it into your mouth determine to eat real food that is good for you and not GMO'd, hydrogenated, deep fried, chemicalized, salted, or sugared. You must determine to eat live food full of vitamins, enzymes, phytonutrients, carbohydrates, minerals, and proteins.

  These are the building blocks for energy which wake up your metabolism. Dead food, packaged edible substances and so-called fast food, are devoid of these nutrients, burden the liver, and move into fat cells. Live food activates fat-burning. Avoid grains, root vegetables and most fruits (except for berries and grapefruit) to get fat-burning activated faster at the beginning of your diet.

- Finally, for permanent weight loss, determine 'the when' you should eat. Midnight is not a good "when" to eat, but mornings and midday are. You must give your body four to six hours to move the food to the large intestines before you go to bed. There are no rules that you must eat breakfast, lunch and dinner.

Even Hippocrates, the father of medicine, said that if you are overweight to only eat once a day.

The old notion that you must eat all day long to keep your metabolism going is falling out of favor to intermittent fasting. If you eat all day long, your body never needs to use the glycogen stored for energy. Try intermittent fasting four days a week to ignite a glycogen (fat) burn. Don't eat for eighteen hours (include sleeping hours.) You can eat two meals the remaining six hours which should include healthy fats, protein, and fruits and vegetables.

When you understand why, what, and when you eat, you don't have to count calories and exercise until you pass out. You will naturally heal your metabolism, lose weight, and feel so much better.

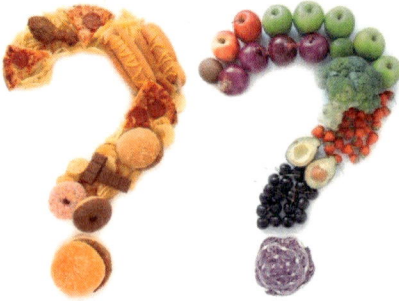

COLOR ME THIN please. I came up with an idea to help my family and clients create a diet that was easy to visualize and remember. I asked them to visualize a plate that contained three-fourths colorful foods and one-fourth white or brown food. The white or brown food consists of proteins and grains that are usually variations of those neutral colors.

The point was to help them realize that a variety of colorful fruits and vegetables was their goal for each meal. If you are looking at your plate and you don't see a rainbow of beautiful colors filling most of it, then you are gaining weight with each mouthful. Like my *Color Me Thin* FB page and get colorful food ideas.

I hope you understand that your body SIZE MATTERS and not just for vain reasons. Your SIZE MATTERS for your health and longevity. For those of you who are overweight, when is the last time you really felt good inside and out?

Throughout this book, there are many ideas about how to lose weight and get healthier.

Come on my beautiful friend, let's live younger, leaner longer!!

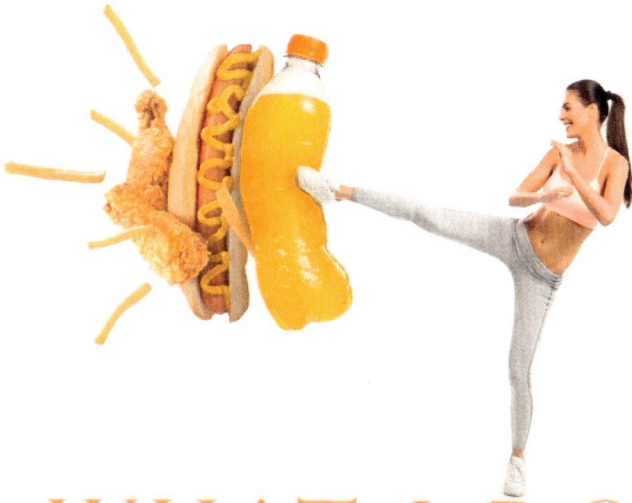

WHAT I DO

1. I buy organic, non-GMO fruits, vegetables, and proteins.

2. I never buy fast food.

3. I start each morning with a fat-burning mixture of one tablespoon of organic apple cider vinegar and one cup of water. You can add another cup of water and the juice of half a lemon also or drink that before lunch.

4. Breakfast is a protein smoothie (with berries, juice of one lemon, half an avocado or nuts, MCT oil, and greens) or protein with good fats (egg cooked in butter.) More about good fats in the chapter STARVATION.

5. When I am trying to lose weight, I do the 18-hour fast during the week. If we have dinner at 7:00 PM, then I only drink liquids until 1:00 PM the next day. I like to add MCT oil to my coffee for extra energy.

6. I cook at least five dinners per week.

7. When we go out to restaurants, I eat veggies and protein and avoid starches and dessert.

8. I collect salad recipes, cook books, and cook from scratch.

9. I grow fresh herbs and hope to add a bed for greens soon.

10. I read labels and avoid products with added sugar like salsas, ketchup, salad dressings, barbecue sauce, tomato sauce, spaghetti sauce, pickles, and relishes.

11. I snack on nuts, seeds, avocados, olives, and occasionally cheese with gluten-free crackers.

12. Stevia and monk fruit are my tea, coffee, and dessert sweeteners (which have no calories and do not affect blood sugar levels).

13. I avoid grains, except for the occasional brown rice, gluten-free pasta, or quinoa.

14. I cook with coconut oil and butter and use olive oil and MCT oil for drizzling and dressings. Good fats don't make you fat.

15. I balance root vegetables with two other vegetables or mixed greens.

16. I follow the Color Me Thin plan and fill most of plate with colorful foods and eat small portions of grains, beans, and/or animal proteins.

17. I realize food is fuel for my body and not fodder for my soul.

Chapter 10

SLEEPLESSNESS

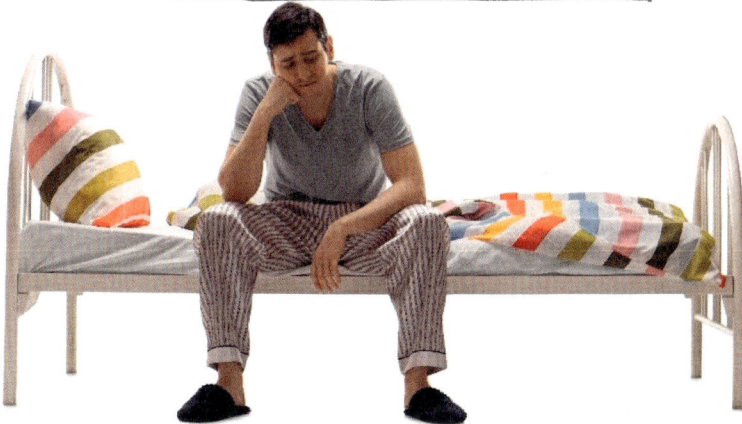

It is estimated that seventy million people have insomnia aka SLEEPLESSNESS. It is fast becoming the number one health problem in America. **Over thirty million people take sleeping pills that have over one million side effects, including mortality.** Sleeping pills suck vital nutrients out of your cells and it takes four and a half years to **cleanse** the liver of these over-the-counter and prescription drugs.

When you don't sleep, melatonin is not released and the mind cannot enter into dream sleep where your memories are consolidated, which is now being linked to Alzheimer's. Dr. Daniel Amen, author of *Change Your Brain, Change Your Body*, has done over seventy-four thousand brain scans. He explains that without at least seven hours of sleep, there is not enough blood flow to the brain for regenerative health and prevention of Alzheimer's.

Without enough sleep, you are more at risk for infection, insulin resistance, obesity, cardio-vascular disease, arthritis, and mood disorders. Your body needs sleep to detox and repair cognitive issues.

According to the horary cycle or circadian rhythm, different meridians in the body affect the energy balance and renewal of vital organs throughout the day and night.

If SLEEPLESSNESS occurs during one of these P.M. periods, your body may need balancing and health concerns addressed. For instance, if you consistently wake up around 3:00 A.M., there may be a problem with your liver or lung meridian.

For the sake of time, I will not go through the entire twenty-four-hour time clock and all the meridians. Please check out the entire clock for yourself, and if you are awake when you shouldn't be and tired during the day when you should be awake, then your body is trying to tell you something.

For now, let's focus on the evening and why you need to make sleeping well as important as eating well if you want to live younger longer. From 9:00 P.M. to 11:00 P.M. your endocrine system adjusts to homeostasis (the tendency of the body to seek a condition of balance or equilibrium within its internal environment) based on electrolyte and enzyme replenishment. Your body wants to cool down and get balanced as the liver begins to store blood.

This is the time you need to wind down and get ready for bed. It is best to be asleep by 10:00 P.M. Between 11:00 P.M. and 1:00 A.M., the gall bladder begins an internal cleansing of tissues, processes cholesterol and enhances brain function. Then from 1:00 A.M. to 3:00 A.M., the liver is cleansing the blood and processing waste. Now, on to the morning and 3:00 A.M. to 5:00 A.M., the lungs begin oxygenation and expulsion of waste gases.

Large intestines need to move between 5:00 A.M. to 7:00 A.M. to make room for nutritional intake. That is why a warm glass of lemon juice when you awake will help stimulate bowels and the lymph system to remove toxins. If you are experiencing SLEEPLESSNESS during any of these time meridians, it's time to get serious about your health and wellness.

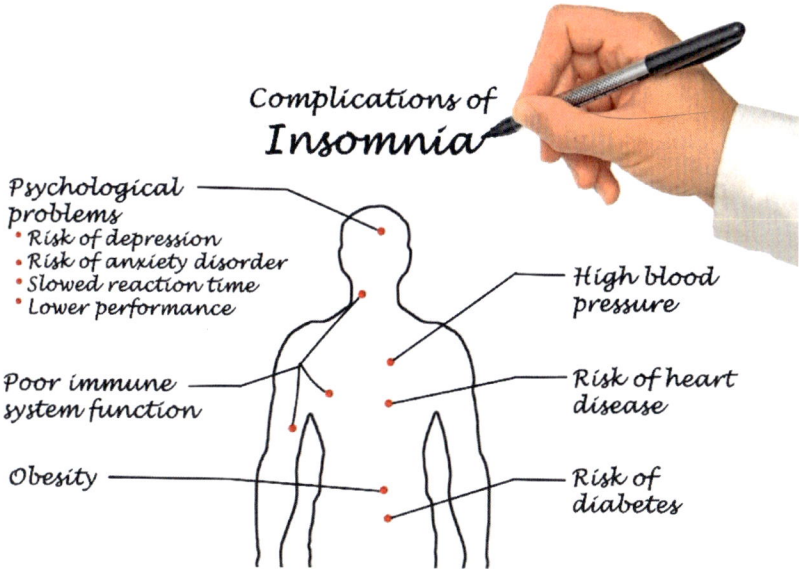

Complications of
Insomnia

Psychological problems
- Risk of depression
- Risk of anxiety disorder
- Slowed reaction time
- Lower performance

Poor immune system function

Obesity

High blood pressure

Risk of heart disease

Risk of diabetes

Apparently, not sleeping makes you fat too! I know, I said that word again. Studies from Christian Benedict and Uppsala University in Sweden show that just a few nights of SLEEPLESSNESS change the gut biome that are the key to maintaining a healthy metabolism. It also causes an imbalance in hormones that promote the feeling of fullness to those that make you feel hungry. The study also shows it affects your sensitivity to insulin. To resist that donut, you need to sleep!

What does lack of sleep do to your skin? Lack of sleep produces cortisol which is called the flight or fight hormone, also known as the death hormone when you can't stop producing it, and you can't stop if you don't sleep. **Cortisol breaks down collagen and**

elastin leading to premature wrinkling. SLEEPLESSNESS shows up on your face in the form of dark circles under the eyes, blemishes, and pale or ashy skin.

According to dermatologists, your skin has to repair at night. During the day, organs like the brain, heart, lungs, liver, etc. are receiving most of the nutrients and oxygen to function properly. Your skin, which is really the largest organ in your body, receives nourishment through the capillary system (the outermost ends of veins which reach the dermis) when the other organs are at rest.

Of course, it's my business to believe your skin is the most important organ in your body. You can remove half your brain and still live. You can remove your uterus, ovaries and spleen and still live. You can replace your heart and liver and even a kidney, but you can't remove your skin and live.

You can patch it here and there but you cannot remove your earth suit and live! So, if you don't get enough sleep, your skin will not get the nourishment it needs to renew and revive itself. With the right amount of rest and nourishment your skin will replace itself every month.

- A word about sleeping naked. There is a growing body of evidence that sleeping naked can have a number of benefits of which sleeping better is one. I began sleeping this way out of necessity because of hot flashes. Other benefits include boosting metabolism, improving blood circulation, balancing hormones, skin and genital health and more. Do your research and see if it is right for you.

- Did you know that employers are advised not to hire individuals who get less than seven hours of sleep because studies show they make too many mistakes?

Establish a regular night time routine for going to sleep. Turn off electronics between 9:00 p.m. and 11:00 p.m. Wear orange glasses to reduce blue light which inhibits your body's production of melatonin. **Do not** keep your phone or iPad next to your bed while you are sleeping at night. Lowering bedroom temperatures helps promote deep sleep.

Sleep.org recommends that bedroom temperature should be between sixty and sixty-seven degrees Fahrenheit for optimal sleep. This produces quality REM (rapid eye movement) sleep which is the stage of sleep with the highest brain activity.

You may need 'white' noise to help you relax. New research from the Northwestern University Feinberg School of Medicine suggests that 'pink' noise, a mix of high and low frequencies that sounds more natural, is better for memory function and repair and a deeper sleep than its cousin 'white' noise. Their patent-pending discovery should be available soon.

Make time for wind down: read, pray, meditate, stretch, etc. Take melatonin or Ashwagandha supplements. Calcium with magnesium aids relaxation.

You need to sleep. Get serious about solving SLEEPLESSNESS so you won't age so fast.

WHAT I DO

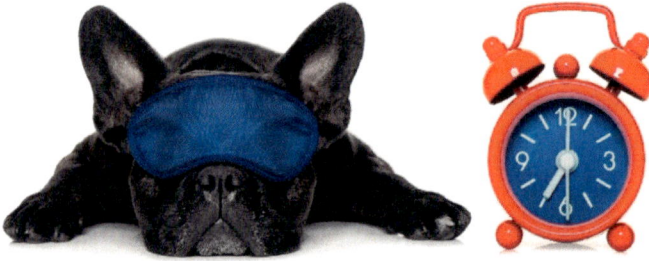

1. I take my calcium/magnesium supplement right after dinner. These minerals promote relaxation and are better utilized by the body when taken in the P.M.

2. I also take Ashwagandha, which is another supplement that is known for its calming effects.

3. I take melatonin supplements while getting ready for bed. It is a powerful antioxidant, anti-inflammatory, and immune builder, even though it is most known for helping regulate the sleep-wake cycle.

4. I use an all-natural progesterone cream. Dr. Amen teaches that it is like valium for the brain.

5. The lights in our house are on timers to turn off at 10:30 P.M. Alexa dims the bedroom lights to ten percent as we get ready for bed.

6. The thermostat automatically drops to sixty-eight degrees at 10:30 P.M. That's as low as I could convince my husband to go.

7. I have an air filter/fan on my side of the bed that not only circulates cool filtered air; it provides a quiet 'white' noise. I really can't wait to get the new 'pink' noise though!

8. I keep an eye mask in my bedside table just in case I want to go to bed early or sleep late. The darker the room the easier it is to produce melatonin.

9. I usually get ready for bed and complete my night facial regimen around the same time every night.

10. If it has been a stressful day, I put HOT towels on my face, shoulders, neck, chest and stomach. (Avoid your face if you have broken capillaries or rosacea).

11. I **sleep on my back to prevent wrinkles** being pushed into my face. This is one of the best ways to save your face. You will need to train yourself, but it can be done. Imagine fifty years of pressing wrinkles into your skin. If you do sleep on your side, push the pillow back and let your face hang off the side. Keep your face away from the pillow!

12. I take my pillow if traveling as often as I can.

Chapter 11

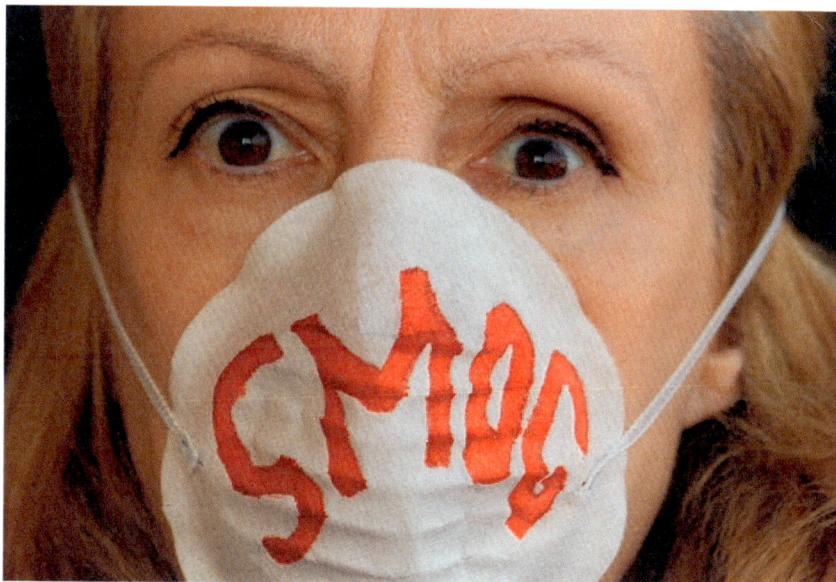

The word SMOG was coined in the early 20th century and is a combination of the words smoke and fog, generally applying to a mixture of smoke and sulfur dioxide resulting from coal burning. Now the definition of air pollution is more sophisticated including a mixture of ground level ozone, sulfur dioxide, nitrogen dioxide, and carbon monoxide. Other components of the SMOG of today are lead, mercury, arsenic, benzene, formaldehyde, pre-retardants, radon, and other volatile organic compounds (VOC's).

According to the WHO, the World Health Organization, air pollution in 2014 was responsible for over seven million deaths. They contend that it is a "greater global threat than Ebola and HIV." Even though air quality has improved in the U.S., around fifty percent of its residents are still affected and are mostly living in California, Kentucky, and Pennsylvania. London has had serious problems lately, and the pictures of cities covered in

SMOG in India, Pakistan, Uganda, and China and around the world are alarming.

No, I am not a tree-hugger (although I love trees) or think the planet is doomed. I just want to bring attention to the sometimes-invisible toxic situation of air pollution and how it affects our aging and longevity. Seniors, children, and people with chronic health issues are at highest risk.

SMOG can not only contribute to premature death, heart disease, asthma, stroke, diabetes, and obesity; new studies link it to depression, anxiety, Alzheimer's, dementia, and poor academic performance. Although research is on-going and filtering out slowly, SMOG not only affects our body, it could also affect our brain.

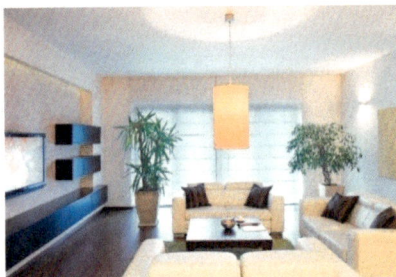

Continuous toxic chemical overload will overwhelm and impair the incredible human immune system. Being aware of the not-so-obvious, sometimes invisible SMOG in your home and your city will help you win the battle on premature aging and chronic disease. Here are a few suggestions for the home, city and the skin.

IN THE HOME
- Test your home for radon emissions (second leading cause of lung cancer), and get a carbon monoxide detector
- Use a vacuum cleaner with a HEPA filter
- Mop or dust with plain water to clean remaining particles
- Look for home improvement materials with low VOC's
- Use water-based paints since they have fewer fumes than solvent-based

- Consider electric or gas fireplaces if you have respiratory issues
- Consider the outgases from furniture, carpet, flooring, and fabrics
- Use door mats to reduce chemicals from coming into your home
- Leave shoes at the door and change into slippers, thongs, etc.
- Do not use plug-in air fresheners (testing found as many as twenty chemicals)
- Use essential oils and diffusers for health benefiting aromatherapy
- Look for naturally scented cleansers
- Use baking soda and lemon for cleaning and/or vinegar and water
- Consider an indoor filter and carbon HEPA air conditioning filters; check air systems once a year
- Keep humidity at 30%-50% to prevent mold and reduce dust mites, and have your house checked for mold
- Make your home a no-smoking zone (smoke contains over 4000 chemicals)
- If your home was built before 1978, you may have lead paint which damages your brain, nervous system, and kidneys.
- Consider indoor plants and a Himalayan salt lamp for assisting with indoor air purification

IN THE CITY

- Check air pollution forecasts daily if you have chronic health issues
- Avoid exercising, walking, or playing outdoors if air pollution or SMOG is high. Instead go to a gym or mall.

- Stay away from high traffic areas
- If you do go outdoors and air quality is poor, wear a mask
- Plan ahead; keep provisions to avoid shopping on SMOG-filled days
- After venturing out in SMOG, shower when you return home

FOR YOUR SKIN

- The skin is a major component of our immune system and as I have said "my favorite organ." Our skin protects us from the environment by keeping bacteria, viruses, and other air-borne pollutants from getting inside.

  The guardian cells in the epidermis include dendritic, phagocytic, and Langerhans cells. They love an acidic pH of 4.5 to 5.5. This acidic mix of surface oils and moisture forms the acid mantle.

  The acid mantle is a very important element of the skin's protection component. It's important to keep your skin clean, but not to strip away this protective layer by using harsh chemically-laden and fragranced soaps.

- Avoid toners or fresheners with alcohol or fragrances also

- Your skin can absorb oxygen, nitrogen, and other air-borne toxins so be aware of this damaging and aging dilemma: SMOG.

Protect the atmosphere in your home or office and you will protect your health. Protect your skin that lives in that atmosphere because it protects you!

Remove the invisible SMOG in your home. If you can see SMOG, protect yourself to protect your health and longevity.

WHAT I DO

1. I have door mats at front and back doors.

2. I leave 'outdoor shoes' by the back door and other shoes in the mudroom.

3. I have HEPA air conditioning filters.

4. I have indoor air filters.

5. I have diffusers around the house and loads of essential oils. Get a desk reference guide to essential oils from *Life Science Publishing*.

6. I use only water to dust and mop.

7. I use perfume sparingly and only spray it on my clothes or a cotton ball.

8. I use all natural aloe vera soap or our Aloe Body Wash for bathing.

9. I use the Hello Gorgeous toners as they have no alcohol or fragrances.

10. I keep a Himalayan salt lamp in the bedroom and the office in our home. These are amazing, but make sure it is made of genuine salt and not a plastic look alike. These lamps are great for air purification.

They attract water vapor in your home that usually comes with air pollutants like mold, bacteria, and allergens. When the vapor hits the lamp, the salt traps the pollutants and releases the vapor.

They also emit negative ions which reduce the positive ones coming from the electromagnetic fields (electrosmog) of electronic devices like cell phones, computers, lamps, televisions, iPads, etc. There are more than two thousand studies that show consistent exposure to electrosmog or low-level radiation cause a "variety of cancers, impair immunity, and contribute to Alzheimer's disease and dementia, heart disease, and many other ailments," explains Dr. David Carpenter, coauthor of the *Bioinitiative Working Group Report* public health chapters.

11. Himalayan salt helps ease symptoms of asthma and allergies. You have probably heard of salt spas or salt caves. The salt lamp helps bring some of these benefits to the home.

The negative ions also help reduce anxiety and promote a peaceful atmosphere helping you sleep better. These ions also increase oxygen to the brain producing "higher alertness, decreased drowsiness, and more mental energy," according to *WebMD*.

12. I live in Texas, way north of Dallas, where there is no industrial SMOG, but the invisible stuff that make allergies go crazy are still there.

Chapter 12

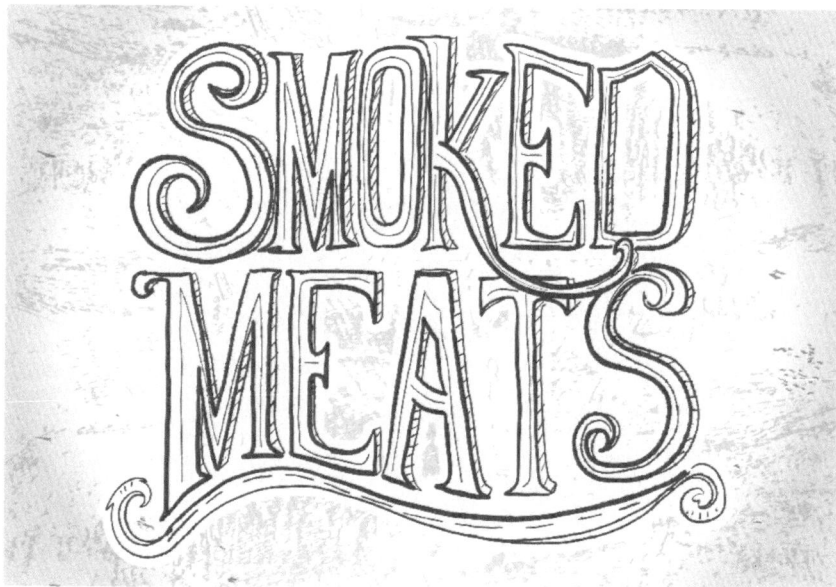

I've never been a big fan of SMOKED MEATS, but if you are, you will want to read this chapter. The flavor of SMOKED goodies is quite scrumptious. Does your mouth begin to water when you think of Applewood smoked bacon, Hickory smoked prime rib, or Mesquite smoked brisket? **Unfortunately, these tasty burnt offerings may be aging you, even killing you.** Even eating burnt fries or toast puts you at risk for cancer according to a recent study in the U.K. by the Food Standards Agency.

So, what's the big deal? Here is a little cooking chemistry 101. When you apply heat to food, a chemical process takes place. Different types of cooking (grilling, smoking, boiling, frying, baking, slow cooking, etc.) produce different chemical reactions producing different tastes of the same food type. When you add spices or marinades, even more chemical reactions take place. As you may surmise by now, some of the chemicals produced during some of these cooking methods are known as **carcinogens**. You can find out loads of information on carcinogens (chemicals that cause cancer) at *cancer.gov* and the National Cancer Institute.

Here are some of the nasty culprits that harm your health:

- Heterocyclic Amines (HCAs) are one of the chemicals formed when MEATS or fish are grilled, SMOKED, are fried at high temperatures. According to a study published in *PubMed,* ten different HCAs have been identified which are highly mutagenic. When fed to rodents, these HCAs, produced cancer in the colon, breast, and prostate. The National Cancer Institute says a diet rich in HCAs is linked to breast, colon, liver skin, lung, prostate, and other cancers. Well done meat has three and half times more HCAs than medium rare meat and fried pork has more than fried chicken or beef.

- Polycyclic Aromatic Hydrocarbons (PAHs) are probably the most infamous of the toxic chemicals created when SMOKED or grilled. PAHs are formed when fat and juices from meats or fish drop on a wood, charcoal, or gas fire and create SMOKE! PAHs are in the SMOKE and then deposit on the protein and your clothing, or in your lungs. According to the American Cancer Society, PAHs lead to skin, liver, stomach, and lung cancer and even leukemia. But wait, it gets worse. When nitrogen from the protein is released during SMOKING or cooking, nitrated PAHs (NPAHs) are formed which are more carcinogenic. Even SMOKE flavorings have PAHs.

- Advanced Glycation End Products (AGEs) are a normal result of metabolism. The problem comes when we cook animal or fish protein with dry heat like SMOKING, grilling, or broiling. This increases the formation of AGEs ten to one-hundred-fold circulating through your body. Also known as glycotoxin, these pathogenic agents are responsible for sponsoring kidney disease, diabetes, atherosclerosis, inflammation, and slow wound healing. High meat diets are responsible for more breast, colon, and prostate cancer. According to the *Journal of the Academy of Nutrition and Dietetics,* animal-derived foods are generally AGE rich and prone to AGE formation during cooking.

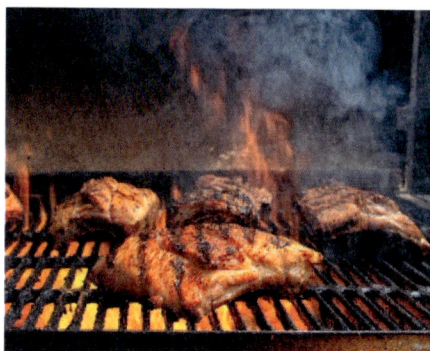

"In contrast, carbohydrate-rich foods such as vegetables, fruits, whole grains, and milk contain relatively few AGEs even after cooking." For more information on diet-related AGEs, please check out the studies on *PubMed.*

No, I'm not telling you to torch your grill.

There are a few things you can do to reduce PAHs, HCAs, and AGEs and therefore reduce adverse effects on your health.

1. Serve more organic vegetables and fruits to serve with your doomsday delicacies, I mean your backyard barbecue. ☺ According to an article in the *Huffington Post*, Mrs. Colleen Doyle (director of nutrition and physical activity for the American Cancer Society), says to make your veggies the star of the meal. Grill as many as you can and get that same hot-off-the-grill flavor says *Health.com.* A good way to do this is to make veggie kebabs.

2. All of you, who order your meat rare, will love this. "Just pat it on the butt and run it across the grill," is how one of my friends puts it. Turns out, rare meat has fewer carcinogens

than well-done meat due to the shorter cooking time. Well-done meat was linked to a sixty percent higher chance in developing pancreatic cancer according to *Health.com*.

3. Squelch the SMOKE on your food and the air you breathe. Remove the skin from chicken and trim the fat from meats. Choosing leaner cuts of meat will help reduce those flaming PAHs, too.

4. Spice it up and reduce toxic HCAs and AGEs by up to sixty to ninety percent. Red pepper, thyme, sage, garlic and rosemary are just a few examples according to *Health.com*. Other good spices that work are black pepper, ginger, cloves, oregano, cardamom, mustard, paprika, onion, and turmeric.

5. Alcohol to the rescue. Never thought I would say that. Beer and wine marinades reduce carcinogens by forty percent when marinated six hours prior to grilling, says *Health.com*. Even if you only have thirty minutes to marinate, it still prevents carcinogen formation says Mrs. Doyle. A lemon juice, onion, and garlic blend will reduce toxicity up to seventy percent. Another great blend is apple cider vinegar and olive oil.

6. Ditch the barbecue sauce says Dr. Joseph Mercola and the *Natural Medicine Journal*. Sauces made with tomato and/or sugars double or triple your ingestion of carcinogenic compounds even after only fifteen minutes of cooking.

7. Lower the heat to 325 degrees Fahrenheit (or below) which is when the toxic chemical reactions start happening. Dr. Mercola recommends that steak should be 145 degrees F, hamburgers 160 degrees F, and chicken 165 degrees F. Use a thermometer for best results.

Traditionally, beautifully choreographed grill marks were the sign of future happiness in your mouth. Now you know, you are just cooking up cancer. Scientists have known about this since the 1960's after a ten-year study was completed in Eastern Europe. They studied countries where their primary food was SMOKED MEATS and fish and the link with gastrointestinal cancers. Thank goodness these and other studies are seeing the light of day so that you can be more aware of what is aging you, even killing you.

If you want to slow down the aging process and stay healthier, you will have to make a few changes in the way you grill and perhaps ditch the SMOKED MEATS. You can still cook up some backyard beauties, now that you know what's happening.

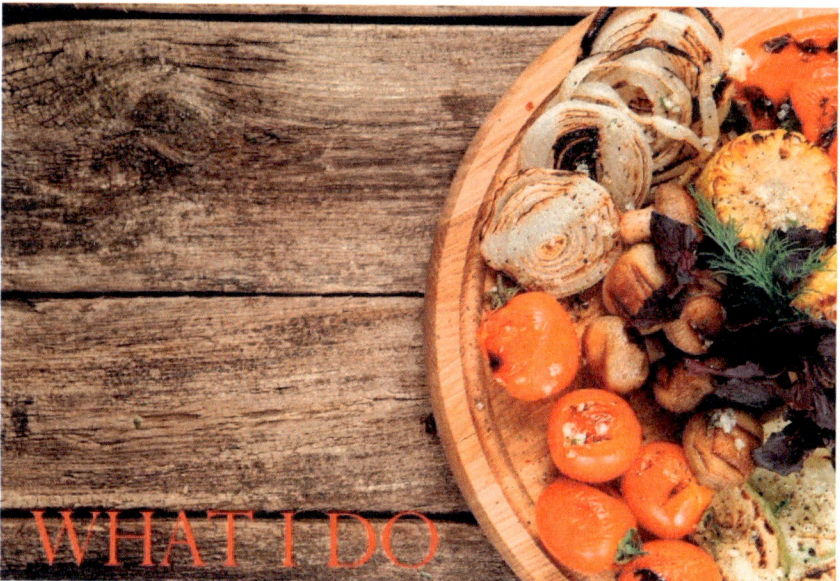

WHAT I DO

1. I love our outdoor living area that has a stove top and a grill. I marinate all the meat, chicken and fish before cooking. For lamb and beef: red wine, lemon juice, crushed garlic, fresh rosemary, and organic Worcestershire sauce.

For chicken: beer, lemon juice, onion, turmeric, and ginger. For fish: lemon juice, lemon slices, fresh tarragon and oregano, minced garlic, and olive oil. All proteins are cooked off flame.

2. I do make veggies the star of all my meals. Please check out some of ideas on my Color Me This Facebook page. One of my favorites is kebabs with bell pepper, tomatoes, onions, zucchini, and snow peas. Sometimes I add small organic potatoes that I pre-boiled.

    When I add mushrooms to kebabs, I sauté them in butter, Worcestershire and soy sauce first. I have a flat stainless-steel cook top that takes the place of a couple of grates so nothing gets burned. Asparagus and root vegetables are grilled on this as well. I cook meat kebabs with only onion and garlic.

3. I always serve a fresh salad when cooking on the grill. I also love to serve melons while we are cooking!

4. I grill corn in the husks (that I have soaked in water) and serve with seasoned butter, flavored cheese, or herbal-chive toppings.

5. Grilled fruit, like pears or peaches, topped with my homemade whipped cream is my family's favorite.

6. We watch the grill temperature and make adjustments when the temperature exceeds 325 degrees F.

Chapter 13

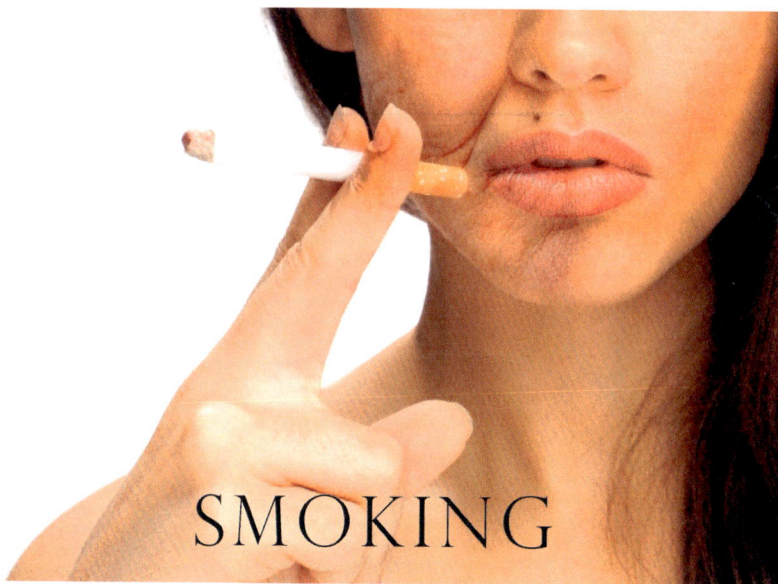

SMOKING

The CDC (Center for Disease Control and Prevention) says that over thirty-six million adults smoke in the U.S. They also report that 3200 youth, under the age of eighteen, light up a cigarette for the 'first' time each day. Each day 2100 youth and young adults become daily smokers. **According to the CDC one hundred eighty thousand deaths occur each year due to SMOKING.**

Not only does SMOKING kill you, it makes you chronically sick. Do I even have to talk about this one? The CDC says SMOKING leads to disease and disability and harms nearly every organ of the body. **It is the leading cause of preventable death.**

According to the American Lung Association it causes lung cancer, COPD (chronic obstructive pulmonary disease), stroke, asthma, reproductive problems in women, premature and low birth-weight babies, diabetes, blindness, cataracts, age-related macular degeneration, and over ten types of cancer including colon, cervix, liver, stomach, and pancreatic. Wait, there's more. Smokers develop a secondary primary cancer as well. This should scare the bejeebies out of you if you are a smoker.

So, it is destroying your insides but just what is it doing to your face? **SMOKING makes you look prematurely old**. OLD before your time, STOP it! SMOKING affects women more drastically because men have more collagen and elastin fibers in their skin than women do. Their skin is thicker and tighter, so wrinkles will show up faster on women's faces over men's faces, which smoke and are the same age. You'll see the smoker lip lines so much sooner girls!

SMOKING clogs the capillary network which carries nutrients directly to the dermis, so the skin does not have the nutrients it needs to encourage cellular production. SMOKERS' skin looks dull, sallow, and gets prematurely thinner.

In fact, SMOKING stimulates so much free radical damage that it depletes the vitamin C in your body which is essential for maintaining collagen and production of collagen. Smokers and former smokers need to double or triple their vitamin C intake and find skin care products that encourage stem cell production and collagen formation like my Collagen C Complex.

SMOKERS should eat loads of vitamin C rich foods like oranges, red and green peppers, kale, Brussels sprouts, broccoli, strawberries, grapefruit, and guava.

All of that is no cure for all the aging damage that SMOKING is doing to you, so STOP IT!!

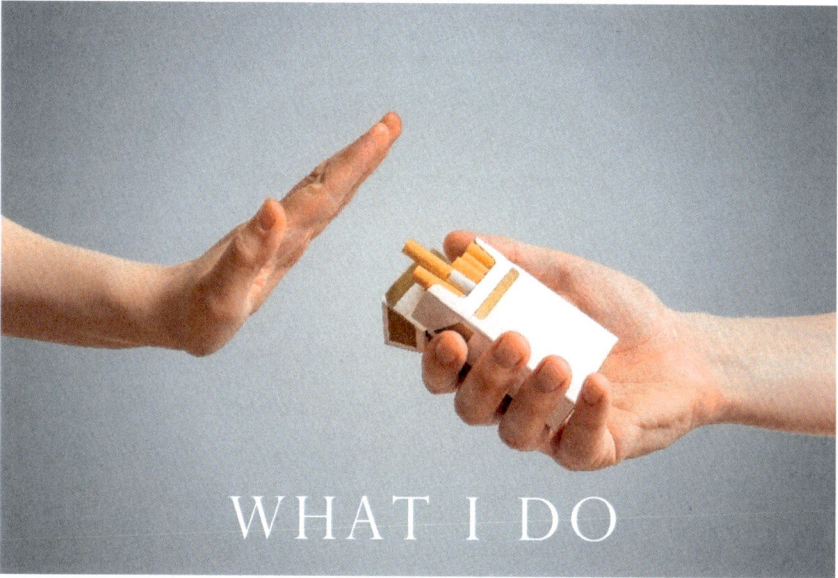

WHAT I DO

1. I don't smoke. I dabbled with it in my thirties, but quickly gave it up when I realized I would get those tiny lines around my mouth that my mother had. She was such a gorgeous young woman, but SMOKING ruined her looks.

2. I do use the Hello Gorgeous Collagen C Complex serum which contains vitamin C, collagen, and Swiss apple extract which stimulates new skin stem cells, promotes collagen production, and reduces age spots to combat aging.

3. I eat loads of salads with dark leafy greens, use peppers in everything I cook practically, put citrus in my smoothies, and eat broccoli and Brussels sprouts several times a month for ample amounts of vitamin C.

Chapter 14

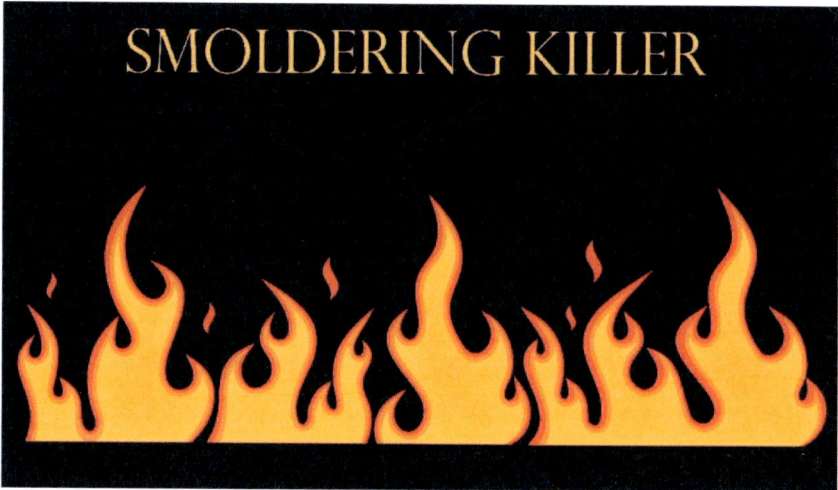

SMOLDERING KILLER

I want to tell you about a SMOLDERING KILLER that is lurking in your body that you probably do not feel or know it exists. **There is a silent war going on that produces no symptoms, usually, until an actual health crisis occurs.** It can predict heart attacks, heart failure, diabetes, becoming fragile in old age, cognitive function decline, and even cancer. Russell Tracy, a professor of pathology and biochemistry at the University of Vermont College of Medicine, says inflammatory factors predict virtually all bad outcomes in humans.

This SMOLDERING KILLER is chronic inflammation. **If you do not stop it, it will be like a weapon of mass destruction in your body aging you beyond your years and ruining your quality of life.** The sad thing is, so many have chronic inflammation and it is preventable.

Not all inflammation is bad for you. Our body has an ingenious way of handling foreign invaders like bacteria and viruses or removing damaged cells. The immune system responds by sending white blood cells and other chemicals to the problem area, and acute inflammation usually lasts only a few days. This is good and necessary inflammation.

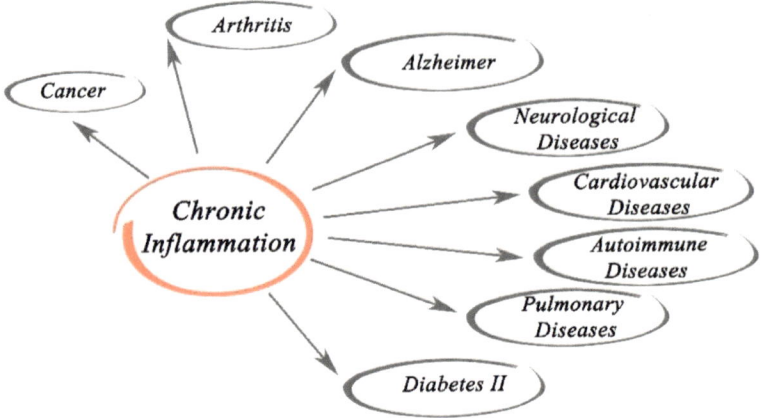

The problem is chronic inflammation, which is when your immune system is sending out a response when no threat is present. When inflammatory triggers are continuously cycled through your blood, they damage nerves, organs, connective tissues, joints, and muscles. "Have you or a loved one dealt with pain, obesity, ADD/ADHD, peripheral neuropathy, diabetes, heart disease, stroke, migraines, thyroid issues, dental issues, or cancer?

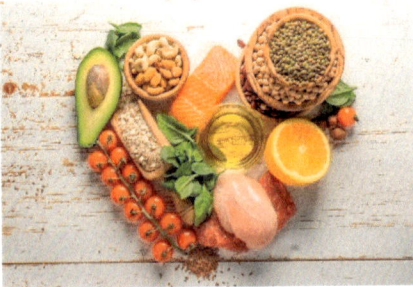

If you answered yes to any of these disorders you are dealing with inflammation," says Dr. David Marquis (board certified in clinical nutrition). Failure to eliminate this constant assault on healthy cells ultimately produces conditions like "asthma, allergies, autoimmune disease, heart disease, cancer, and other diseases, depending on which organs the inflammation is impacting," explains Dr. Joseph Mercola.

Since diet is probably the biggest culprit, I will give you a few easy solutions to eradicate chronic inflammation for good. It's really pretty simple and the food is fresh and delicious.

Foods and fluids are the fuels that make you tick or make you sick.

Here's a great plan for an **anti-inflammatory diet**:

- Eliminate sugar and high glycemic foods (pastry, pasta, potatoes, white rice, white bread, candy, cookies and sweet drinks.)

- Avoid all trans fats: hydrogenated or partially hydrogenated oil that are found in margarines, crackers, breads, vegetable oils, coffee creamers, and most packaged foods, mixes, and sauces.

- For omega-3 support eat avocados, walnuts, pecans, hazelnuts, almond butter, free-range eggs, and ground flaxseed.

- Season food with turmeric, ginger, curry, garlic, onion, cinnamon, rosemary, thyme, cloves, sage, Jamaican spice, marjoram, and Italian spice. New studies show that ounce for ounce, they have more antioxidants than fruits and vegetables. Turmeric, ginger, and rosemary are highly effective at inhibiting inflammatory triggers.

- Consume cruciferous vegetables four times a week which includes broccoli, bok choy, cabbage, cauliflower, mustard greens, and Brussels sprouts.

- Drink green tea every day. The catechins reduce inflammation.

- Add berries (blueberries, strawberries, raspberries, and cherries) daily to smoothies, desserts, topping yogurt, or just eat them. Pineapple is also effective as it contains bromelain, a natural anti-inflammatory agent.

- Add peppers (hot and sweet) to your diet four times per week to salads, sauces, soups, and sautéed with vegetables.

- Alliums like garlic, scallions, onions, and leek should be eaten four times per week.

- Cook with coconut oil and MCT oil and drizzle olive oil every day.

- Add dark chocolate to smoothies and coffee daily.

- Beans (black, red, white and navy), and fish (salmon, sea trout, mackerel, tuna, black cod, herring, anchovies, and sardines), and chicken (free-range) are the anti-inflammatory proteins for this diet.

- Limit red meat (grass fed) to once a week and avoid processed meats.

- Colorful root vegetables (beets, carrots, turnips, and sweet potatoes) should be eaten three times per week.

- Other important fruits and vegetables are grapefruit, apricots, red grapes, tomatoes, apples, spinach, okra, eggplant, and dark green leafy vegetables.

- Eat fermented vegetables to optimize gut flora: kimchee, miso, kefir, natto tempeh, pickles, sauerkraut, olives, and mixed vegies in glass containers.

- Whole grains like oatmeal, brown rice, quinoa, and bulgur should ONLY be eaten three to four times per week. Avoid wheat, rye, and barley.

- Red wine is the preferred alcoholic beverage on the anti-inflammatory diet.

Dr. Mercola says your diet probably counts for about "eighty percent of the health benefits you reap from healthy lifestyle choices," so just cooling down your diet will go a long way in reducing chronic inflammation. By adding a few supplements and making a few changes in your daily routines, you can almost nip this in the bud.

- Insulin resistance is explained in great detail in the SUGAR chapter. Apparently, it is the worst of the worst health problems you can have because it promotes silent, chronic inflammation throughout the whole body. Dr. Ron Rosedale, a specialist in nutritional and metabolic medicine, **says that insulin resistance is the basis of virtually all chronic diseases and the most significant marker for lifespan.** He says that the two key factors in preventing insulin resistance are avoiding sugar/fructose and grains (whether in drinks or food) and performing regular exercise.

- The **'omegas'** are probably one of your best anti-aging/anti-inflammatory nutrients that can help you prevent the SMOLDERING KILLER that plagues most humans today. You need to understand their importance as they must come from outside sources since your body cannot manufacture them from the food you eat. In other words: you have to eat them. The problem is the imbalance between omega-3s and omega-6s in the diet.

Both of these omegas are necessary for survival, but when there are excessive omega-6s consumed compared to omega-3s, there is inflammation. Omega-6s are found in corn oil, soybean oil, sunflower oil, poultry, some nuts and seeds, and just about every pre-packaged food in the grocery store. Some reports say the average American eats a ratio of 12 to 1 and as much as 25 to 1, omega-6s to omega-3s. The proper ratio should be no more that 4 to 1 (anti-aging experts prefer 1 to 1). Without enough omega-3s, your body turns omega-6s into arachidonic acid which is highly inflammatory.

- You can see why inflammation is rampant and a change in your diet is necessary, as well as, supplementation with this anti-inflammatory superstar. The *Journal of the American College of Nutrition* recommends EPA and DNA omega-3s from fish because they are more "biologically potent" than ALA omega-3s from plant sources. The *American Journal of Clinical Nutrition* reports that clinical trials revealed women with the highest intake of omega-3s, compared with women with the lowest, had a forty-four percent reduced risk in dying from inflammatory disease.

- To get more omega-3s in your diet eliminate processed oils like soy, corn, canola, cotton seed, sunflower, and safflower. Cook with coconut oil, MCT oil, and olive oil. Add more wild-caught salmon, mackerel, swordfish, albacore tuna, white fish, and sardines; and grass-fed beef and lamb to your diet plan. Chia seeds, flaxseeds, walnuts, and hemp seeds can be added to smoothies, desserts, and cereals.

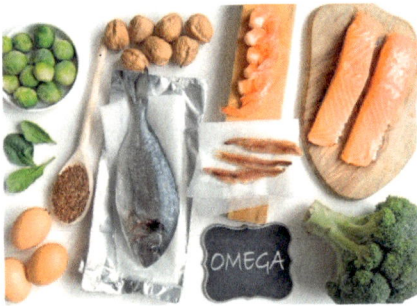

The best omega-3 vegetables are Brussels sprouts, kale, spinach and watercress. Eliminate all packaged foods, mixes, and cereals that contain hydrogenated or partially hydrogenated oils.

Many health professionals recommend salmon oil, cod liver oil and krill oil supplementation to fill in the diet gaps. Make sure your omega-3 supplementation contains EPA, DHA, and zeaxanthin for best results.

- I know some of that was repetitive, but I hope you can see the connection between food and inflammation. Other important anti-inflammatory and anti-aging superstars are:

1. Resveratrol is one of my favorites. It's found in cocoa, certain fruits like grapes, and some vegetables. It is found in abundance in red wine and in this form is more easily absorbed. Resveratrol can cross the blood-brain barrier and has the ability to control certain molecules that trigger inflammation. Studies have proven that it increases the lifespan of cells.

2. Astaxanthin is a powerful anti-inflammatory anti-oxidant that is found in microalgae or sea critters that eat these microalgae like salmon, shellfish, and krill. It is a carotenoid and is what makes fish pink or orange. It is more powerful than vitamins A, C, and E. In fact, it is the most powerful anti-oxidant known to man which suppresses a variety of inflammatory mediators and protects against free radical damage to internal organs. I love this stuff!

3. Vitamin K2 is an important vitamin that works with Vitamin D. It is found in natto, brie and Gouda cheese, and some fermented vegetables. Dr. Cees Vermeer, a top K2 researcher, recommends 45 mcg to 185 mcg daily. Vitamin K2 prevents inflammation by inhibiting production of monocytes in white blood cells.

4. Boswellia, also known as Frankincense, contains active anti-inflammatory agents. I love this oil.

5. Vitamin D is another important vitamin most everyone is deficient in, so get tested every year. Most people need to supplement but the SUN is the best source of Vitamin D.

Read the SUN chapter for more information on how to increase your exposure.

6.   Exercise is one of the most important things you can do to reduce chronic inflammation. Yes, you should walk more and fitness trackers will keep you on your toes (seven to ten thousand steps a day). Read my chapter on SITTING if you have a desk job to understand how SITTING is slowly killing you and what to do. If you have serious inflammatory issues, high intensity interval training (HIIT) interspersed with plenty of recovery time will produce faster results than less strenuous exercise. Over exercising will do more harm than good, though, so seek out good advice.

7.   Sleep is also important, so read my chapter on SLEEPLESSNESS and get more sleep to calm down inflammation.

8.   Grounding or Earthing is proving to be a great way to distinguish the fires of inflammation. Please read my chapter called SHOES AND SNEAKERS to learn more about this fascinating new science.

9.   STRESS sends an endless supply of cortisol into your blood stream which ignites the fires of inflammation that are never distinguished. More information on how to dowse those flames in the chapter on STRESS.

This silent SMOLDERING KILLER, chronic inflammation, often goes unnoticed until serious damage has occurred somewhere in your body. To stay ahead of the game, ask for two tests that can indicate inflammation when you get your annual checkup: 1) C-Reactive Protein (CRP) test, 2) ESR (sed rate) test.

Don't let this SMOLDERING KILLER ruin your chances to live younger longer. You only get one life to live. I think that used to be a soap opera. Oh well, you know what I mean.

Take care of that earth suit you live in, and don't let chronic inflammation steal your creativity and your productivity which puts the joy in living!

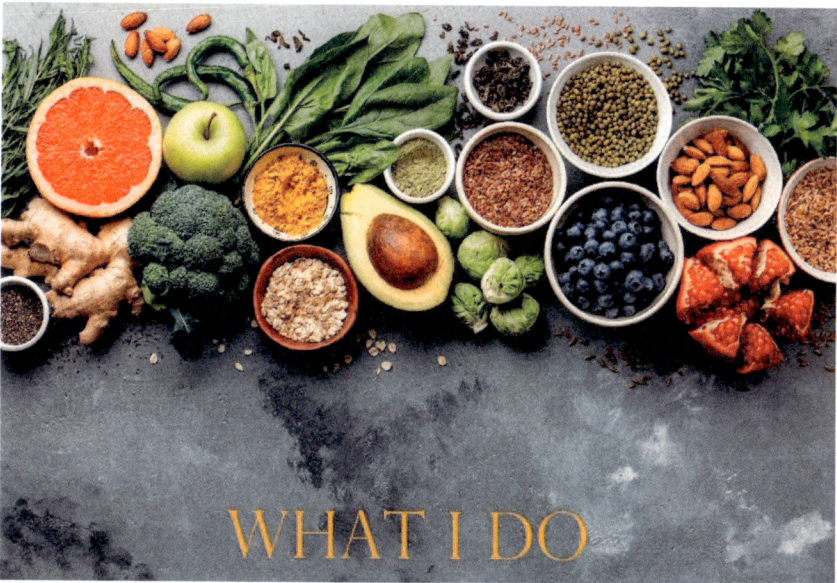

WHAT I DO

1. I make sure that the meals I prepare follow the anti-inflammatory diet.

2. I cook with loads of spices, especially in stir-fries and soups.

3. I eat a bowl full of berries just about every night.

4. I quit using SUGAR probably 20 years ago. I have never really been that fond of desserts and pastries, so it was easy to give up. Not too long after that I discovered stevia.

5. A few years ago, I adopted a gluten-free protocol as well, avoiding wheat, rye, and barley.

6. I drink red wine and a little white wine. I have never been a big fan of mixed drinks or sodas that contain loads of sugar.

7. I drink green tea throughout the day.

8. I use the elliptical instead of the treadmill to get my steps in. Of course, with my job, I stand and walk a lot.

9. I have a full-body vibration machine, hand weights, and resistance bands that I use several days a week. I use yoga for core strengthening and my yoga mat is grounded.

10. We are adding a pool to the back yard for more grounding, de-stressing, and fun with the grandkids!

11. I have a grounding mat under my desk to place my bare feet on when SITTING.

12. I sleep seven to eight hours every night so my brain can detox, reset, and rejuvenate.

13. Even though we eat really well, I still take supplements. I have always felt that the older you get, the more anti-oxidants you need. I take resveratrol, co-enzyme Q10, Astaxanthin, EPA and DHA omegas, turmeric, vitamin C, vitamin D, L glutathione, and zeaxanthin with lutein.

Chapter 15

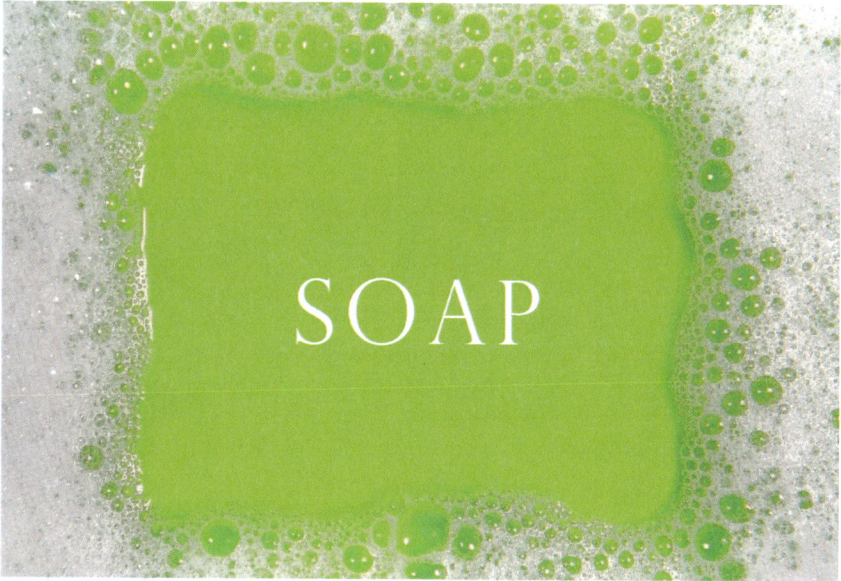

SOAP

Who knew that cleansing your face, washing your hair, cleaning your house, or brushing your teeth could age you?
My goal here is to bring awareness to SLS (sodium lauryl sulfate) because there are over sixteen thousand studies which mention its toxicity. SLS is a surfactant, a substance that breaks up surface tension by breaking the bonds between molecules in the outer layer of a compound resulting in producing lather.

This same surfactant is found in garage floor cleaner, as well as, toothpaste! Many studies reveal cellular DNA damage and digestion problems if ingested. That is why there is a warning on toothpaste containers about not swallowing toothpaste. The *International Journal of Toxicology* recommends that products with prolonged use (such as toothpaste) contain SLS at no more than one percent. Some cleaning products contain SLS levels as high as twenty percent to thirty percent. The American College of

Toxicology has found that even concentrations of less than one percent can cause skin irritation.

Here's the main problem: protein denaturing. <u>When exposed to SLS, a chemical structure forms a bridge between the fat and water-soluble portions in cells reducing its ability to heal itself.</u> When protein is damaged, the body tries to heal the distressed cells, but over time the construction of new cells is diminished and the destruction of cellular tissue is irreversible.

To add more bad news, SLS can become contaminated with dioxane which is a suspected carcinogen and remains much longer in the body because the liver cannot metabolize it effectively. Also, TEA (triethanolamine) is in most shampoos (and skin care products) and when combined with SLS it forms a nitrosamine which is a known carcinogen.

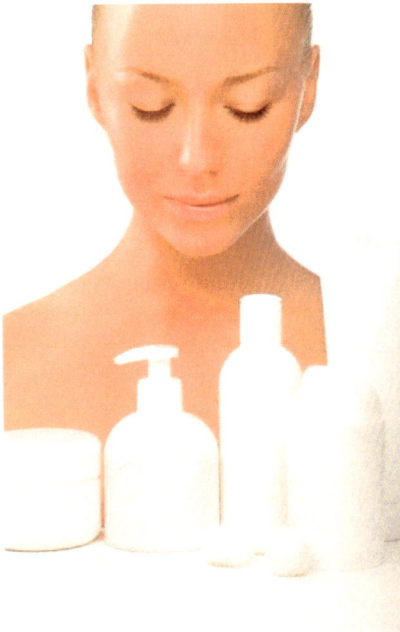

Accounts vary, but women add as much as TWO HUNDRED chemicals daily to their skin and sixty percent reach the bloodstream. Several studies show SLS will remain in a person's system (brain, heart, and liver) for up to five days.

You can see that it never leaves your system with repeated use of house hold cleaners, detergents, shampoos, body and facial products, and toothpaste. It is estimated that you will absorb almost five pounds of chemicals and toxins into your body each year. "This toxic load can become a significant contributing factor to health problems and serious diseases, especially if your diet and exercise habits are lacking," says Dr. Mercola. There are many experts, including Dr. Doris Rapp, that detail the adverse effects of SLS and many other chemicals on our health and our offspring. Please check out their findings.

All that, just to say this: "SOAP can age you." Learn to read labels and avoid products with triethanolamine and SLS. Simplify your life by using less personal care products or using natural alternatives. Look for natural bath soaps made from olive oil, goat's milk, and aloe vera. Always wear gloves when cleaning your house, car, or business. Use a gentler dishwashing liquid.

Be aware of your surroundings and all the ways you come into contact with chemicals. I have only focused on SLS, but the personal care industry is a fifty billion-dollar industry which does not scratch the surface of the home and industrial cleaning industry. There are chemicals everywhere that could affect your health and ultimate age you. **No, I am not a crazy fanatic, but I am aware of these offenders and try to eliminate or avoid them as much as possible.**

Avoid Chemicals like these:

A word about **FLUORIDE**: If you want the whole scoop about fluoride, check out the documentary: *Fluoride, Poison On Tap*. It will scare the bejeebies out of you. Fluoride, as you know, is found in toothpaste and municipal water systems, but what you don't know is that fluoride is toxic. You may not know for decades it was used to reduce thyroid function because it causes cell death.

That is why you are not supposed to swallow the toothpaste, yet, they pump it into the water supply and want you do drink it. Exposure to fluoride causes skeletal fluorosis (weak bones), calcification of cartilage (arthritis), thyroid toxicity, infertility, kidney disease, and inhibits neural development in children (lowering their IQ) according to Dr. Edward Group.

Recent studies at Harvard have classified it as a developmental neuro toxin as published in *Lancet Neurology*. There is a movement and lawsuit filled that will finally end the farce of the benefits of fluoride for tooth decay prevention. According to the National Oral Health Conference, 57 percent of America's youth have dental fluorosis (mottled and discolored enamel). According to Dr. Dean Bark (co-founder of the National Cancer Institute), fluoride causes bone cancer.

I could go on and on, but I think you get the picture. If you want to slow down the aging process, get a home water filter and stop buying toothpaste with fluoride in it.

A word about **PARABENS**: Parabens are commonly used as preservatives in skin care, cosmetics, deodorants, shampoos, soaps, drugs, and food additives. Parabens have estrogenic-like properties and have been found in ninety-nine percent of breast cancer tissues sampled. Enough said, read labels and avoid these chemicals: methyl paraben, propyl paraben, isobutyl paraben, ethyl paraben, butyl paraben, and E216.

A word about **DEODORANTS**: I confess, I do not use deodorant. I learned about this harmful underarm juice years ago from holistic guests on my radio show. Studies reported in the *European Journal of Cancer Prevention* show that women who used deodorants with **ALUMINUM** tend to have higher rates of breast cancer.

The function of aluminum in deodorant is to plug up pores to keep you from sweating and to also kill bacteria. However, aluminum tends to kill the good bacteria and leave the ones that cause odor (basically defeating the purpose). Other ingredients in deodorant include parabens and phthalates (preservatives for fragrances that are toxic to reproductive glands, the brain, and lungs).

Another problematic ingredient is **TRICLOSAN** used to kill bacteria in SOAP and many bath and beauty products. It has been linked to hormonal disruption, impairing thyroid function, and possibly brain development. Another problem is fragrances with **PHTHALATES**. They are used in just about everything but have ingredients concealed due to trademarks.

You are better off rubbing a lemon or lime under your arm (or use the Hello Gorgeous Aloe Citrus Toning Mist). Other safe solutions include a spray made with vinegar and water or hydrogen peroxide (one teaspoon) in eight ounces. Dust a little baking soda under your arms with a ball of cotton or make your own deodorant with tea tree or frankincense essential oils and coconut oil.

I'm not sure plugging up sweat pores with aluminum to prevent perspiration is that good for your health. You need to sweat a little. Tackling the odor is possible with natural solutions that won't age you. A poor diet, stress, health issues, and even deodorant can increase odor causing bacteria. Avoid aluminum and chemically-laden deodorants for better health and longevity.

SOAP and many other additives to the products you use on daily basis are possibly aging you. If you want to live younger longer, you will have to start reading labels and use products that are phyto-based, SLS-free, and paraben-free.

Look for natural alternatives for home-care and personal-care use, to win the war on pre-mature aging.

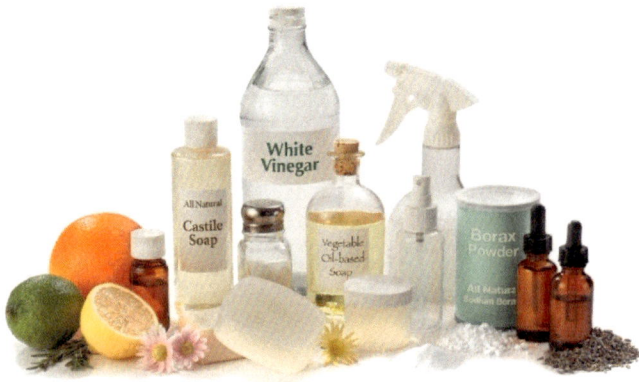

WHAT I DO

1. I wear gloves when doing cleaning chores and working with chemicals at the salon.

2. I use the Hello Gorgeous Aloe Citrus Toning Mist as my deodorant to avoid aluminum.

3. I use the Hello Gorgeous Shea Butter Cleansing Cream for facial cleansing. None of the HG Cleansers have SLS.

4. I clean counters and floors with water only most of the time.

5. I use the Loma hair products from my salon since they are made with aloe and are sulfate-free. You can find them at *hellogorgeous.com.*

6. For body moisturization, I use our Aloe Body Lotion and Coconut Oil which are free of parabens.

7. I always read labels and look for sulfate-free and paraben-free products.

8. I look for environmentally-friendly cleaning products.

9. I use magnetic balls for washing clothes and natural enzyme stain treatments.

10. I use our Aloe Body Wash for showering and Himalayan and Epsom salts for soaking.

11. I use a natural bristle brush for dry skin brushing. Skin brushing encourages circulation and lymphatic flow and is a must for anti-aging!

12. I shop for local goats' milk soap with essential oils at farmer's markets.

13. I never spray perfume directly onto my skin; just my clothing and I use it sparingly.

14. I use natural room sprays around the house from health food stores.

15. We use natural alternatives for all lawn and gardening treatments to avoid harmful chemicals.

16. We have sheep skin rugs to stand on in our bathroom. The natural wool feels wonderful and the sheep skin keeps us grounded.

Chapter 16

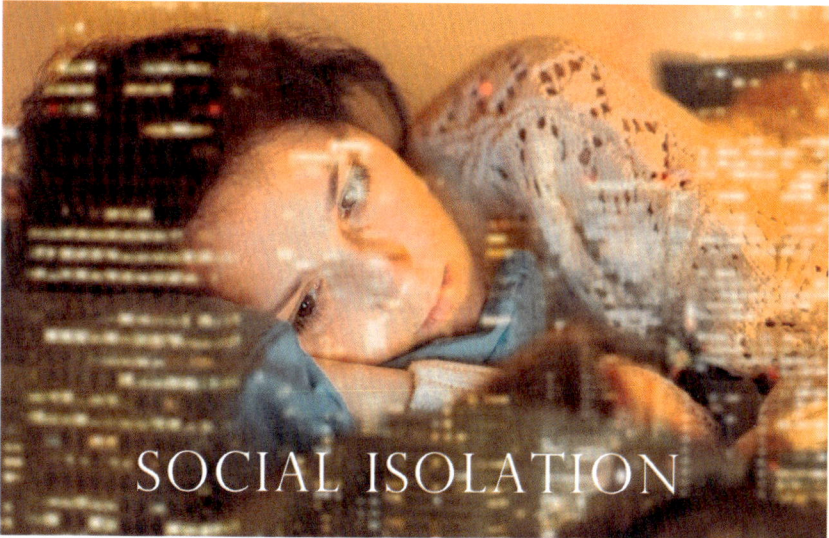

SOCIAL ISOLATION

This chapter collects a few thoughts on SOCIAL ISOLATION or maybe better described as loneliness. In 2015 Brigham Young University (BYU) published its research on the health risks associated with social isolation and loneliness and found that **SOCIAL ISOLATION increases your risk of death by an astounding thirty percent and some estimates were as high as sixty percent.**

In fact, they concluded that loneliness might be a more important risk factor than obesity, smoking, exercise, or nutrition. In 2017, *Forbes Magazine* published an article: ***Loneliness Might Be A Bigger Health Risk Than Smoking Or Obesity***. The article explained that in the last decade there is overwhelming evidence that "a lonely person is significantly more likely to suffer an early death than a non-lonely one." Other associated issues are depression, anxiety, dementia, substance abuse, and even schizophrenia.

While all lonely people are not suicidal, all suicidal people are lonely.

Just the way STRESS negatively affects the body and suppresses the immune system, Doctors are now finding the same physiological impact on the body with SOCIAL ISOLATION. **Studies show that the lonely "suffer from higher all-cause mortality, higher rates of cancer, infection, and heart disease."**

The *Bible* puts it this way, "It is not good for man to be alone." Scientists will tell us that we have a better chance at survival in a group whether family, social, or work, than we do in SOCIAL ISOLATION.

In our Integrative Nutrition training, we learn the importance of 'primary foods' which include spiritually, career, physical activity, and relationships. One of the most important 'primary foods' is relationships. We teach our clients that this 'primary food' is just as important as broccoli.

Nonfood sources can nourish your body on a deeper level than food. Unfortunately, according to the professors at BYU, we are at the highest recorded rate of living alone across the entire country and they are predicting a possible loneliness epidemic in the future.

It's ok to say you are lonely. An AARP survey finds that almost half of Americans experience some degree of loneliness. They have a support group called *Connect2Affect.org*. *Psychology Today* offers ten ways to ease the pain of loneliness:

1. Don't blame yourself in any way, shape, or form
2. Seek relief from a non-human friend like a pet or a great book
3. Connect with a human friend who has always been supportive
4. Do something creative like a puzzle, needlework, or painting
5. Help someone in need, a single mom or an elderly neighbor

6. Find someone else who is lonely and help them

7. Visualize being at a great place like a sporting event or a beach

8. Treat loneliness like a visit from an old friend, it takes away the sting

9. Remind yourself that tomorrow will be a new day

10. Sing your favorite song

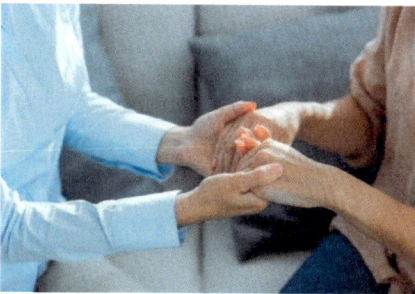

Find a nearby church or synagogue and get involved. Let your family know how you are feeling. Keep in touch with old friends. Volunteer even when you don't feel like it. Clean up a local park. Start a vegetable garden or grow herbs on your kitchen window seal. Volunteer at the local animal shelter. Visit nursing homes or hospital waiting rooms. As much as I love social media, it doesn't take the place of you getting out of your comfort zone and doing something you have never done before or doing something you used to love to do.

Have you heard of hug therapy? Scientists tell us that hugs have hormonal effects on the body, even comparable to the effects of some drugs. The power of touch begins in the womb, to being held as a baby and does not go away as an adult. Some scientists say it even increases as we get older since we don't typically get hugs on a daily basis. When you hug, it gives an instant feeling of closeness and reduces the stress of loneliness and even heals feelings of anger.

Scientifically speaking, hugs stimulate the production of oxytocin, which calms the nervous system, promotes positive emotions, and slows down heart rate. Hugging also helps balance white cell production because it stimulates your thymus gland (hugs keep you young). Babies who were hugged a lot have less stress as adults. Seniors who are hugged lose the fear of loneliness and death.

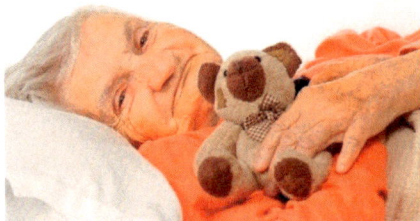

Hug a Teddy: I was really touched by a study done by the Vrije Universiteit Amsterdam. The study, published in the *Journal of Psychological Sciences*, revealed that even hugging an inanimate object like a teddy bear can sooth existential fears. Sander Koole, lead researcher, said that we are aware we are going to die, but those with self-esteem issues feel their life is meaningless. Hugging instills confidence and helps cope with their fear of mortality. So why don't you save those old teddy bears and other stuffed toys and bring them to a nursing home nearest you?

Finally, a new study published in the journal *Scientific Reports*, analyzed the health data of almost three and half million Swedes. **The study showed that the thirteen percent who were dog owners tended to live longer and were at lower risk of dying from heart disease.** They concluded that dog owners lived longer because dogs provide a social connection and motivation to get out and be more active. Especially important was the fact that single dog owners had a thirty-three percent reduction in risk of death. If you are lonely, please consider a dog. After all, they are "man's best friend." SOCIAL ISOLATION can destroy your health and cause premature death.

I hope I have inspired you to get a friend and be a friend and break the curse of loneliness. You were created to love and be loved. It starts with you.

WHAT I DO

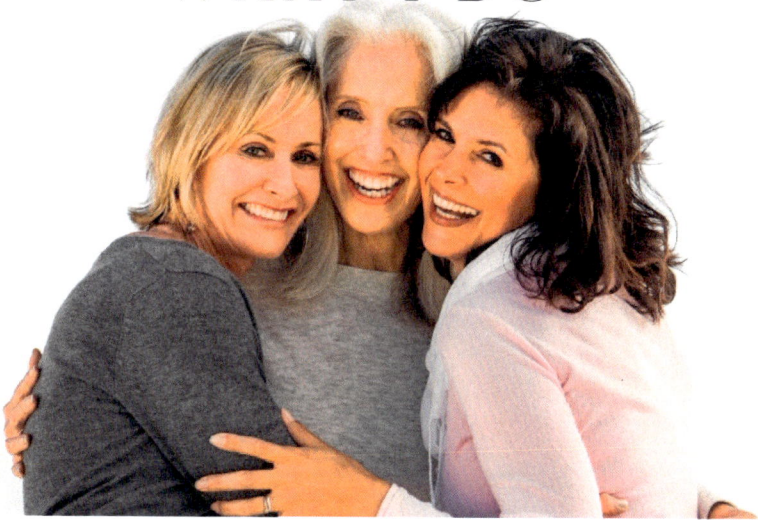

1. I love a girls' night out every now and then. Even a girls' trip is good for the soul.

2. When my hubby is out of town, I go to my daughter's house or make plans with a friend for dinner.

3. I love my dog, Merlot. Yes, that is his name. He is always there for me.

4. I attend many networking groups, and usually find one good connection to build a new relationship.

5. I go shopping or get a pedicure.

6. I have a ritual once a week of scanning magazines for the latest fashion and beauty news.

7. If I'm really feeling down, I just cry, feel sorry for myself, and then get over it. ☺

8. If I know someone is alone, I invite them to church or one of the many networking groups I'm involved in.

9. My team and I go to nursing homes to brighten the lives of the seniors with a day of beauty where we style hair, do makeup, and take pictures! It turns into a day of hugs and smiles all around!!

10. I love to hug my clients and the elderly.

11. I think grandchildren give the best hugs!

Chapter 17

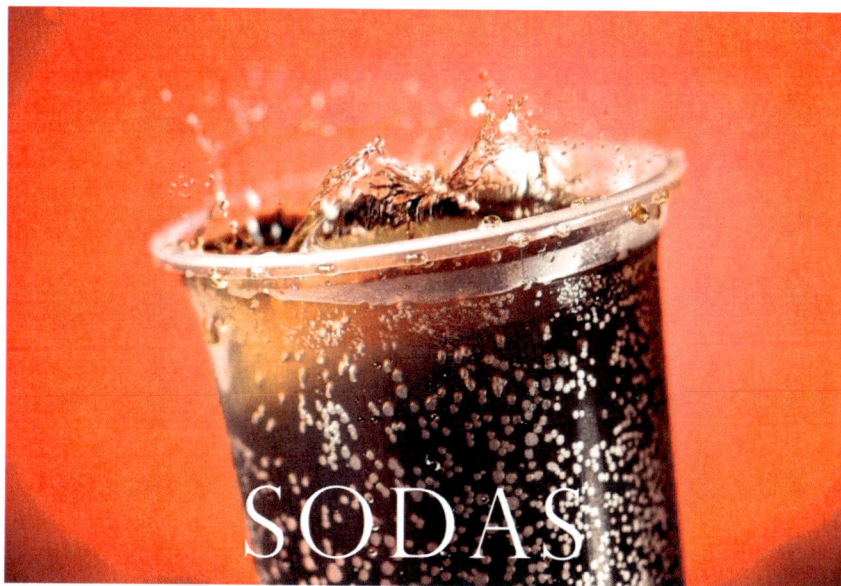

The consumption of SODAS has doubled since the 1960s. In the U.S. alone, fifty billion liters of SODAS are consumed each year which is around **fifty-seven gallons per person**. The National Cancer Institute, the American Diabetes Association, Harvard, *Web MD*, and the book *Sweet Deception* are just a few sources for the latest research on **SODAS causing metabolic syndrome, heart disease, diabetes, obesity, tooth decay, cancer, osteoporosis, non-alcoholic fatty liver disease, and gout.** There should be no doubt that SODAS are stealing your youth and aging you.

SODAS contain ten to twenty teaspoons of SUGAR in the form of high fructose corn syrup. Fructose is processed in the liver and is basically sent into fat storage. Just two cans per day will cause you to gain a pound a week.

SODAS are the number one source of calories surpassing white bread. **Daily SODAS increase the risk of metabolic syndrome by thirty-six percent and type 2 diabetes by sixty-seven percent compared to non-soda drinkers.**

- WHAT IS METABOLIC SYNDROME? It is estimated now that over 75 million people have Metabolic Syndrome. This means that your body is resistant to insulin because of a diet high in starches and sugars. The pancreas cannot create enough insulin to control the rise in blood sugar, so cells stop responding and the pancreas becomes exhausted. If your waistline is not half your height in inches, you probably have it.

- WAIST NOT WEIGHT! The quick new way to find out if you are at risk for heart disease, high blood pressure and diabetes is to measure your waist. British researchers analyzed three hundred thousand people and found this 'new' ratio to be a better prediction of health issues.

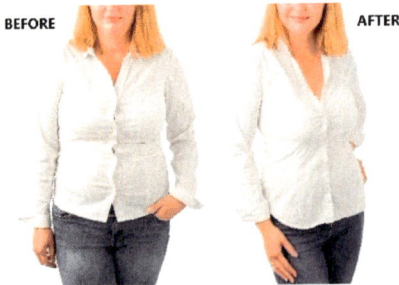

BEFORE   AFTER

Calculate your height in inches and divide by 2. Ideally, if your waist measurement is not less than half, you are at risk. Dr. Margaret Ashwell, who spearheaded the study, says, "Keeping your waist circumference to less than half your height can help increase life expectancy for every person in the world."

- I'M SHRINKING! As we age, our skeletal frame naturally shrinks to some degree as we experience bone loss. For those who have been addicted to this bubbly brew, you have accelerated this aging process. The phosphoric acid in

SODAS inhibits calcium retention and causes bone softening and shrinking, aka osteoporosis.

This leads to the shrinking skull! What happens to the skin on the face of a shrinking skull? It sags, loosens, hangs and falls. A $30,000 facelift can 'nip and tuck' it! Or you can just quit drinking SODAS now!

Healthy treatments like exercise programs with weights, and dietary adjustments, including extra calcium and vitamin D help reverse the bone loss damage. Eating lots of dark green leafy vegetables that provide vitamin K will help prevent calcium being leached from your bones.

Do not think the SUGAR-FREE beverages that soda manufacturers are promoting are a healthier choice. According to *draxe.com*, they are even more deadly due to all the side effects of the artificial sweeteners:

- Diet SODA drinkers are three times more likely to develop dementia and stroke.
- Diet SODAS cause brain damage resulting in poor memory and smaller brain volume.
- Diet SODA drinkers over the long term lose thirty percent kidney function.
- Diet SODAS (four cans a day) put you at thirty percent risk of depression.
- Diet SODAS stimulate cravings for real sugar because the brain identifies the artificial SWEETENERS as fake sugar.
- Diet SODA increases your risk of developing asthma and COPD symptoms.
- Diet SODA drinkers are more likely to suffer heart attacks and strokes.
- Diet SODA drinkers are more likely to die from heart disease.

- Diet SODA drinkers (two or more a day) had a 500 percent increase in waist size over non-drinkers.

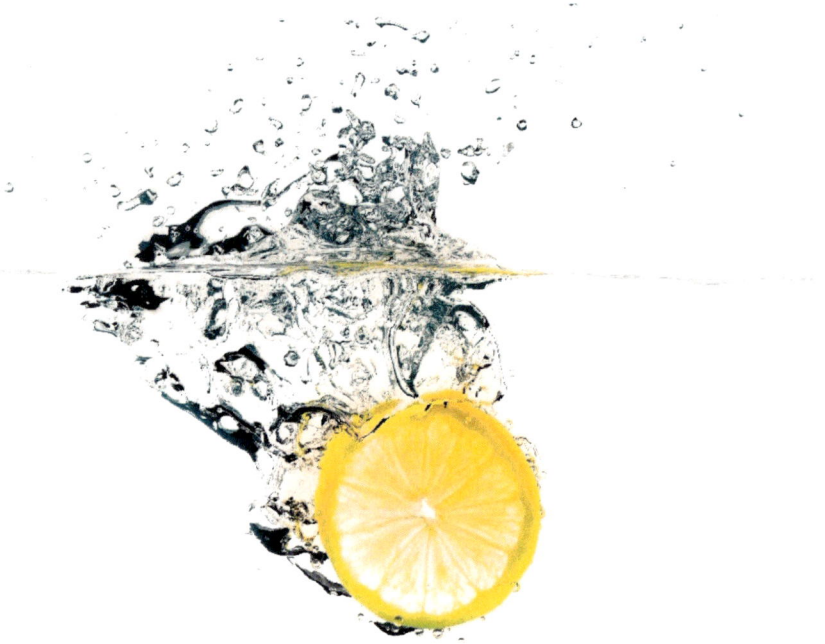

Try naturally carbonated mineral waters to help satisfy your cravings. Drinking more water (with lemon) will help crowd out the need for the sugary potions. Eliminate SODAS and learn to love lemon water! Here is what a glass of water with half a lemon juiced can do for you:

1. It provides natural electrolytes (potassium, calcium and magnesium).
2. It reduces joint pain.
3. It helps the liver produce more enzymes than any other food.
4. It releases toxins from the liver.
5. It regulates bowel movements.
6. It reduces anxiety and depression with its high potassium content.

7. It cleanses the blood.
8. It lowers blood pressure by as much as ten percent.
9. It aids unborn babies in the formation of bones and nervous system.
10. It helps dissolve kidney, pancreatic, and gall stones and calcium deposits.
11. It helps weight loss by curbing hunger cravings.
12. It helps tooth pain and gingivitis.
13. It helps prevent cancer and other diseases by producing an alkaline environment in the body.

Learn to love tea: green, white, and oolong because they contain catechins. These anti-oxidants fight inflammation which is the root of most disease, especially arthritis. Tea lowers the risk of Alzheimer's by up to eighty percent.

Hibiscus tea is becoming the new sweetheart of the tea brigade. According to Web MD and others, hibiscus tea lowers blood pressure, calms the nervous system, reduces inflammation, and improves immunity. The anthocyanins in this tea kill cancer cells and it is found to reduce the risk of stroke and heart attack!

Another alternative to SODAS are the new 'vinegar waters.' They are naturally flavored and slightly carbonated and healthy for you!! Another healthy sweetheart is Kombucha! Naturally carbonated mineral waters with lemon give you a bubbly fix.

You'll find more about tea and its calming effect in the STRESS chapter.

Eliminate SODAS and find healthy alternatives if you want to live a longer, healthy life

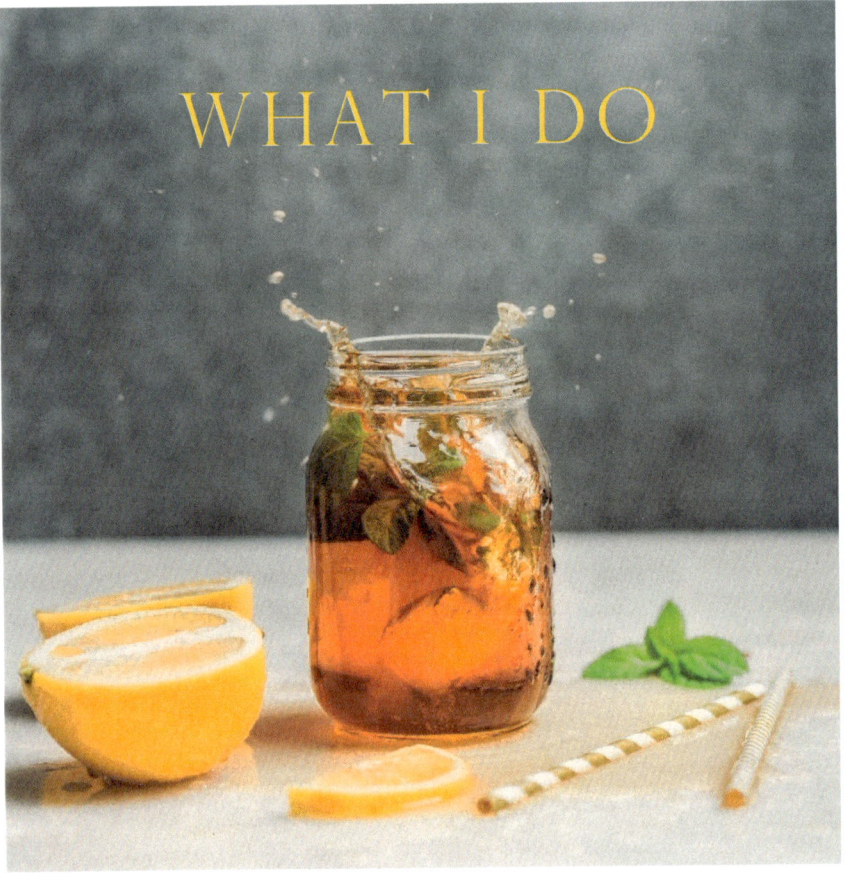

WHAT I DO

1. I drink loads of green tea. I make a big jug every morning and drink it all day long. I add lemon and sometimes mint that I grow on the patio.

2. I drink loads of filtered water with lemon or Fiji water.

3. If I want a change, I buy bottled mineral water, still or naturally carbonated. They even have flavors now. I'm experimenting with flavored vinegar waters as well.

4. I avoid tap water in restaurants. I usually bring my own water (Fiji).

5. Not all water is equal as you know by now. I use a Berkey Water Filter that sits on the counter. It filters out even the arsenic. (I love them so much, I sell them also.)

6. I make spa water with organic cucumbers, mint, blueberries, lemons, oranges, grapefruit, strawberries, etc.

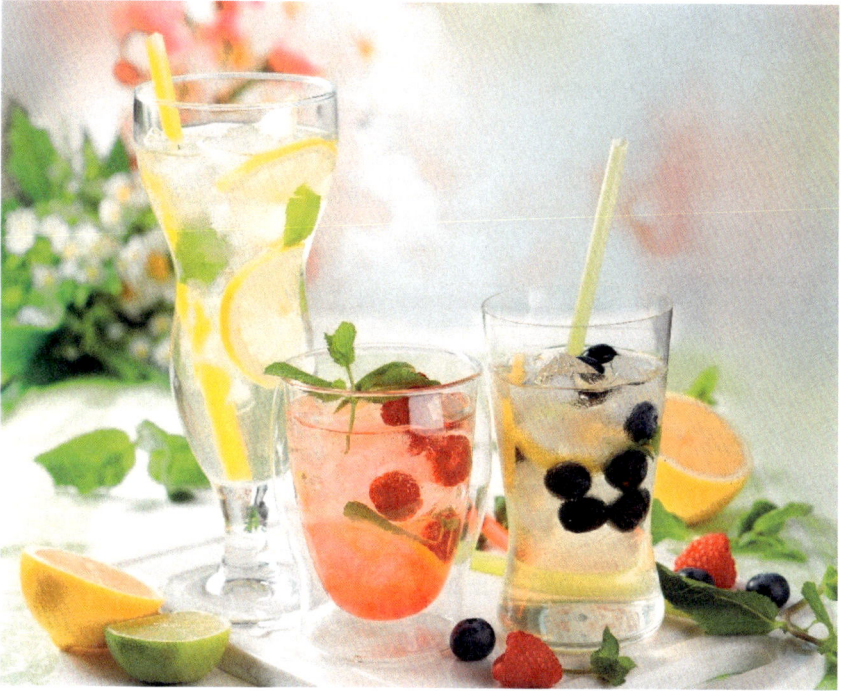

Chapter 18

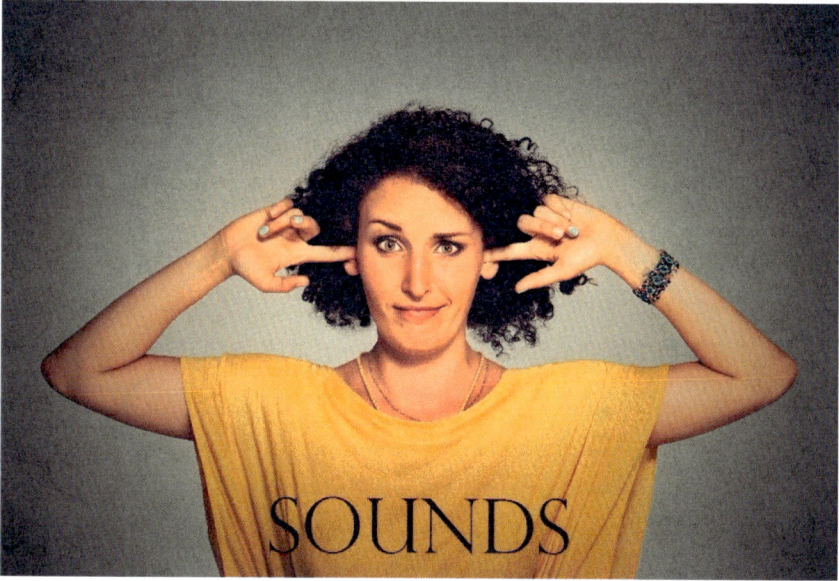

Life in the big city may be making you deaf and even killing you! According to *Medicalpress,* living in a noisy city increases your risk of hearing damage by sixty-four percent. Wait, there's more. *Science Daily*, which reports the latest research news, says: "Your risk of heart attack increases with the amount of traffic noise to which you are exposed." No matter where you live, you can't escape SOUNDS, but some noise is more hazardous to your health than others. **You may be surprised how SOUNDS are aging you.**

Loud SOUNDS were a way to activate adrenalin in our ancestors so that they would be able to fight or flee when they heard the roar of the king of the jungle. Bart Kosko, Ph.D., author of *Noise,* says "we regularly get similar stress hormone surges from car alarms, ringing phones, police sirens, leaf blowers, jack hammers, and amplified voices."

Adrenalin and cortisol constantly rushing into the blood stream causes brain damage, cardiovascular problems, and respiratory issues. **You were not created to be in a constant state of panic.**

Harper's Bazaar Magazine recently had a great article called: *How City Noise is Slowly Killing You.* They cited a study presented to the World Health Organization declaring "noise pollution the number two threat to public health, after air pollution." Arline L. Bronzaft, Ph.D., has studied noise pollution for over thirty years. She explains that, "Even if you don't have health problems yet, you'll have diminished quality of life."

It is the prolonged exposure to SOUNDS registering over eighty-five decibels (dB) that is the problem. An occasional concert at one hundred twenty decibels or a noisy restaurant or bar at ninety decibels may not permanently damage your hearing. However, what if you are employed there? If so, you will need to use protection. Being exposed daily to subway noise and shouting (ranging from ninety to ninety-five dB) and heavy traffic (ranging from eighty to ninety dB) is eventually going to be a big problem for city folks.

Don't think that wearing a personal music device is the answer, since it slams your ears with one hundred dB. If you do choose that route, turn the music down, way down. Many people must endure the constant barrage of loud city SOUNDS, which to some is music to their ears. When in harm's way, though, you really should wear ear plugs.

Have you ever screamed inside your head, "I just need a little peace and quiet!"? Well, you probably do. Your ears never go to sleep, because in part, they were created to help you survive. So, your ears will always be hearing something.

According to a study published in *The Lancet*, exposure to occupational, environmental, and social noise poses a serious threat to public health.

You cannot escape SOUNDS. It doesn't take a rocket scientist to know loud noise can permanently damage your hearing. Now, more and more studies are revealing the effects that all sorts of noise have on sleep, learning abilities in children, high blood pressure, and cardiovascular disease.

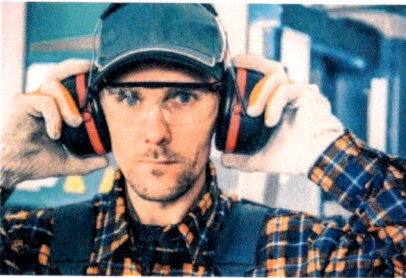

Fortunately, many businesses are aware of occupational hazards and require their employees to wear ear protection, but some may still be behind the times.

Here are a few jobs that are hazardous to hearing according to *Medical Daily*:

- Carpenter: Nail guns (110 - 140 dB)
- Ambulance Driver or EMT: Sirens (110 - 140 dB)
- Lumberman: Chainsaw (110 – 140 dB)
- Musician or Rock Star: Concert speakers (110 – 140 dB)
- Air Traffic Controller: Jet engine (110 – 140 dB)
- Garbage Worker: Truck (85 – 100 dB)
- Construction: Jackhammer (85 – 100 dB)
- Landscaper: Power mower (85 – 100 dB)

For all you NASCAR lovers, one car at full throttle is 130 dB. Imagine forty-three NASCARs at full throttle racing around a track with their SOUNDS echoing off aluminum grandstands. You should wear ear plugs at the very least, but I would recommend investing in decent earmuffs.

According to the American Speech-Language-Hearing Association, approximately forty-eight percent of adults in the U.S. report experiencing hearing loss. **The National Institute of Deafness and Communication Disorders (NIDCD) reports that thirty to fifty million Americans are exposed to dangerous noise levels each day.**

While prolonged exposure to noise registering between seventy to ninety decibels can cause increased hearing loss, even one single loud noise like a gunshot at one hundred and fifty decibels can permanently damage hearing.

It's time to wake up and hear the noise. Be aware of how SOUNDS are affecting you and take precautions. You should not be exposed to more than eighty-five decibels (even when wearing protection) for more than eight hours. Seventy-five decibels or under is preferred in a working environment. The higher the decibels, the less time of exposure you should experience.

SOUNDS are everywhere and they could be slowly and consistently aging you by destroying your hearing and your health. Once those auditory cells are dead, they cannot regenerate.

There is no cure for hearing loss, there is only prevention. Now that you know that SOUNDS can increase your risk for heart attack or stroke, it's time to protect your ears to protect your longevity.

If you want to live younger longer, be aware of the dangers of SOUNDS and get serious about saving your hearing!

WHAT I DO

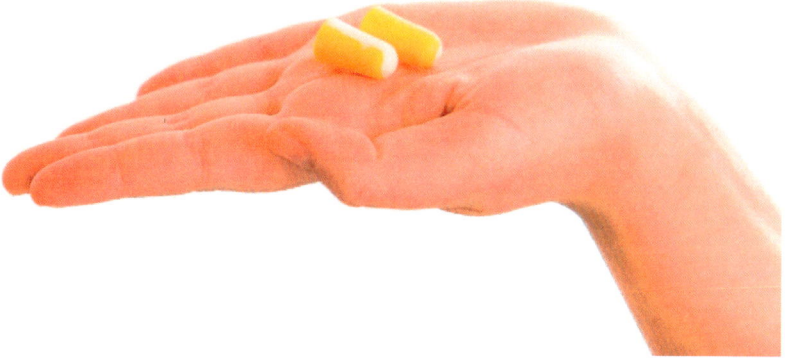

1. As you may have guessed, I don't go to rock concerts. We do go to other concerts, though, but we are not on the front row or near the speakers.

2. I live outside the big city of Dallas, in a small town on a quiet golf course.

3. I work in a small salon with only the occasional noise of a hair dryer or two.

4. I do keep ear plugs in my purse. You never know when you might need them.

5. We wear earmuffs when shooting our guns. Who knows, I may bring them with me the next time I go to the big Apple. ☺

Chapter 19

SOY

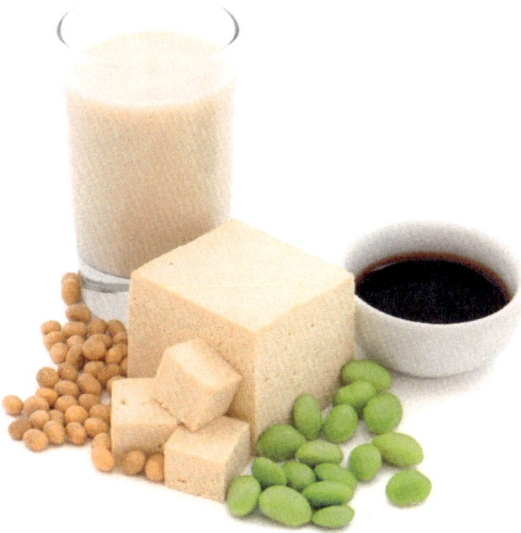

Is SOY the healthy alternative for meat protein or dairy products? **You would think so since forty billion dollars of SOY was sold last year.** SOY milk and tofu is proudly served on vegan and vegetarian tables every day, but are they getting the best bang for their buck nutritionally?

Since ninety-three percent of SOY is genetically engineered, I doubt it. Since many of its components do more harm than good, I doubt it. SOY is not a healthy alternative for those seeking a healthy lifestyle and is probably aging you as you will see.

Let's take a walk down memory lane to the Chou dynasty (1134-246 BC). SOY is one of the ancient grains mentioned during that time and even earlier, but was basically used for crop rotation because of its nitrogen-rich nodule roots. It was considered unfit for human consumption by most cultures. The discovery of soy fermentation occurred during the Han dynasty (206 BC – 220 AD) which enabled them to turn soybeans into a paste and then to soy sauce for food preservation and flavoring meals. **It was found that after months of fermentation, the anti-nutrients were neutralized and digestion was possible.**

Prince Liu An is credited with the discovery of making cooked bean curd into a solid-molded state and thus tofu was born. Some theorize that Buddhists monks or the Mongolian tribes of northern China invented tofu. Tofu was introduced to Korea and finally reached Japan around the eighth century AD. Tofu and fermented SOY foods spread to surrounding regions and eventually tempeh and natto evolved as condiments. Japan is credited with creating miso.

Let's fast forward to 1913. SOY was listed as an industrial product by the US Department of Agriculture, not as a food. Even in Asia, 1930, SOY was still only used as a condiment according to K. C. Chang, editor of *Food in Chinese Culture*. It was only 1.5 percent of their total food consumption.

By 1960, Soy processors discover a way to remove the protein to create SPI (Soy Protein Isolate). By 1999 after millions of dollars are poured into research, the US Food and Drug Administration approved a health claim that 25 grams of SOY protein may reduce the risk of heart disease. **The marketing gurus took the ball and ran with it and turned the simple soybean into a health food superstar.**

Farmers are brainwashed into thinking they can grow the perfect food, a virtual miracle crop that can save the world. *The Furrow*, a magazine written in 12 languages by John Deere, encouraged its readers to plant more of the new health food. SOY manufacturing plants sprung up everywhere to suck out the protein and crush out the oil of the tiny beans extracted from their fuzzy little pods.

From 2000 to 2007 over 2700 new foods containing SOY were introduced and by 2009 over eighty million acres of SOY were planted.

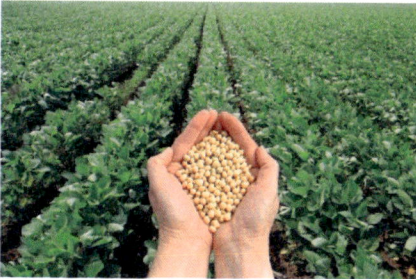

So good was the propaganda that the SOY limits at schools were lifted despite the allergy concerns. It is now in just about every pre-packaged food and salad dressing, and found in too many baby formulas. It is even in corn tortillas and bread.

So, what is the problem? Unfermented SOY, eaten in small amounts, is not really the problem. The problem is that SOY protein and SOY oil are in thousands of products and therefore consumed in much larger amounts than the human body can digest and assimilate.

SOY is one of the top eight food allergens and because of that it is required that it must be clearly stated on every label according to the *Food Allergen Labeling and Consumer Protection Act*.

There are over 170 studies listed on *westonaprice.org*, dating from 1950 to 2013, which describe the detrimental effects of SOY to human health. Some of the findings point out: phytates in SOY prevent mineral absorption, goitrogens block thyroid hormones and iodine metabolism, hemagglutinins cause blood clotting, phytoestrogens promote breast cancer and alter menstrual cycles.

SOY has enzyme inhibitors, which block enzymatic action that breaks down protein which leads to amino acid deficiencies. SOY contains toxic levels of aluminum and manganese due to the exhaustive processing. **Shockingly infants fed SOY formulas have 20,000 times the amount of estrogen circulating in them as opposed to infants fed other formulas.**

Dr. Kaayla Daniel, author of the *Whole Soy Story*, reveals thousands of studies linking SOY to:

- Breast cancer
- Brain damage
- Infant abnormalities
- Fatal food allergies
- Immune system breakdown
- Reproductive disorders
- Kidney Stones
- Infertility
- Digestive problems

If that is not enough, over ninety percent of the SOY crop is genetically modified (GM) which comes with its own set of problems. There is enough evidence to doubt the health claims of SOY, some of which are being challenged and debunked. If the lobbyist and spin artists can keep this from you, they will. It's just not worth the risk when there are so many alternative choices available.

Remember, fermented SOY does not carry the dangers of its unfermented cousin. Enjoy tempeh, miso, natto, and soy sauce if you are not allergic to SOY. Look for organic and non-GMO varieties. One of the benefits of fermented SOY is vitamin K, the forgotten vitamin. It is necessary to prevent osteoporosis, cardiovascular disease, leukemia, and dementia. Vitamin K also partners with vitamin D to help protect you from lung, prostate, and liver cancer.

Skip the tofu, soy milk, soybean oil, soy cheese, soy ice cream, soy yogurt, soy meat (or texturized vegetable protein also known as TVP), soy protein powders, infant formulas with soy, and EDAMAME! Ouch!

You will have to avoid processed foods and stick to fresh, whole foods as much as possible. Always read the label and the small print. Finally, avoid soy lecithin which is found in a myriad of foods, supplements, and skin care.

If you want to live younger longer, you will have to stay away from SOY and its derivatives. Do not think of it as a health food, but rather a fake food!

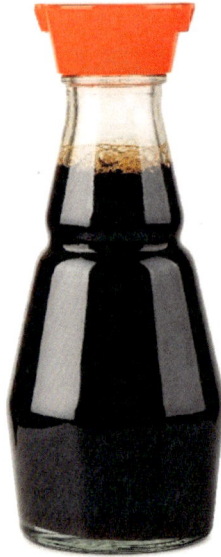

WHAT I DO

1. I use almond milk or coconut milk in my smoothies, cereal, and desserts.

2. I cook mostly from scratch, but otherwise, I am obsessed with reading labels.

3. I have never been a big fan of SOY, but like you probably, I did try tofu to help stretch my protein in casseroles. I soon learned of the questionable health effects from one of my nutritional guests on my radio show, and never dabbled again.

4. I make sure my soy sauce is organic and non-GMO.

Chapter 20

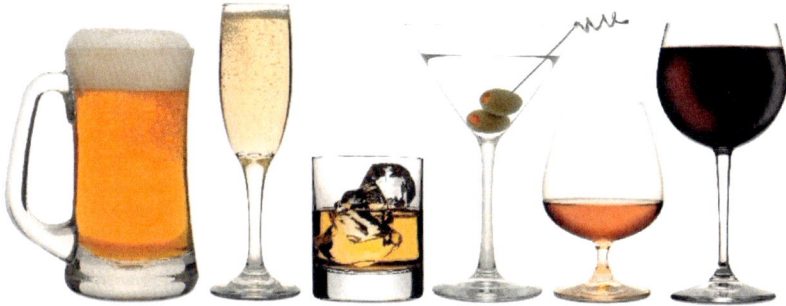

SPIRITS

No, this is not about things that go 'boo' in the night. It's about alcohol consumption, aka SPIRITS, and how it affects the aging process. There are about ninety thousand deaths that occur each year due to alcohol poisoning erasing an average of thirty years off those lives according to the Centers for Disease Control and Prevention.

Women are more prone to alcohol poisoning than men due to their weight, hormonal factors, and the inability to break it down due to less liver enzymes. They also report that one in six adults binge drinks four times a month, which means they consume around eight drinks per binge. Six people die every day from alcohol poisoning.

According to *PubMed.gov*, deaths related to alcohol and cancers have increased by sixty-two percent in the last decade. Cancer in the rectum, liver, colon, esophagus, oropharynx, and breast cancer are associated with alcohol consumption. The CDC reports that in America, the total cost of drinking too much (illness, injury, missed work, etc.) is estimated to be almost 249 billion dollars.

OK, I don't want to be a party pooper, but there are a few things you should know to help you live younger longer. I know you know that too much drinking is not good for you, just like too much eating is not good for you. In this chapter, I just want to break it down a little and let you know why too much alcohol can be dangerous, what it is doing to you, and give you a few suggestions that can help you navigate this sometimes-controversial topic with the least amount of damage.

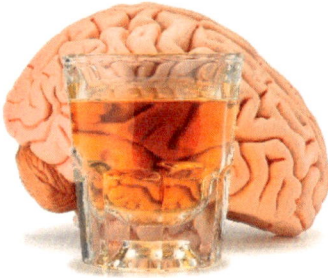

By now, everyone knows that too many SPIRITS can damage your liver, but did you know it will make your BRAIN SHRINK? The National Institute on Alcohol Abuse and Alcoholism reports that the loss of brain volume resulting from heavy, long term drinking leads to dementia in the elderly. Apparently, alcohol causes the Hypothalamus to shrink, which affects your thinking, memory, and learning. No matter what your age, the ethanol build-up prevents the formation of memories, which causes you to forget what you have done. "Did I do that?'

SPIRITS are both a depressant and stimulate, altering brain chemistry, which could confuse a normal person. It usually does. While it can increase dopamine (by exciting the feel-good reward center) for a while, it also affects neural pathways that decrease brain-activity and energy level. You are happy one minute, then tired and sleepy the next.

I'm just skimming the surface, but other aging problems that SPIRITS cause is increased inflammation, heart cardiomyopathy, arrhythmias, high blood pressure, and stroke. It affects your gut biome increasing risk of leaky gut and impairs your immune system. All that is bad enough, but what is it doing to your skin?

According to Dr. Perricone, "alcohol contains destructive molecules called aldehydes, which wreak havoc within your body." **These aldehydes cause cellular damage to** the **plasma membrane and portions of the cell's interior.** SPIRITS, especially mixed drinks full of SUGAR, ignite inflammation which directly affects the largest organ, the skin. It changes the way blood flows to the skin.

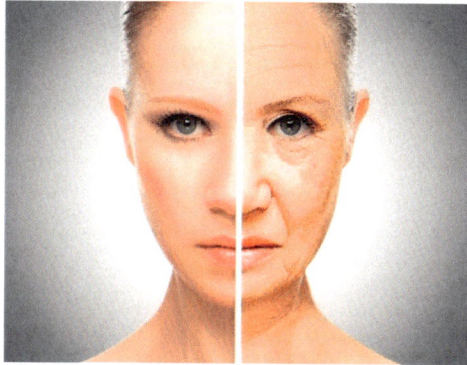

Alcohol widens capillaries which allow a rush of blood to the skin causing flushing and redness. **Over time, the delicate vessels become permanently damaged or broken.** Nutrients and oxygen are unable to reach the skin and a myriad of aging affects are permanently etched onto the facial surface.

Skin problems are also caused by damage to the liver. Alcohol is a hepatotoxin according to Dr. David Colbert, dermatologist. **This is a toxin to the cells that detoxify your body**, he explains in a *Huffington Post* article. "One way to look at it," Dr. Colbert said, "is to ask what does someone look like who is dying of liver failure? They're sallow, they're pasty, they're cold, and their pores are huge."

Ever wonder why you go to the bathroom so much when you drink? Turns out alcohol hinders the production of vasopressin which is an anti-diuretic hormone. This makes the kidneys work harder to remove excess water and sends it to the bladder instead of distributing it throughout the body to all your organs, including your skin.

So basically, you are tinkling away all those important nutrients and fluids you need to stay hydrated and healthy. Your body is about two-thirds water, but if you break it down further, you are about ninety-nine percent water molecules.

So, you can see how this can affect the texture of your skin if it is dehydrated. **The skin collapses leaving it thin and cracking like the Sahara Desert.** Over time, permanent wrinkles, uneven skin surface, enlarged pores, paleness, purple veins, sagging, and blotches result from the lack of nutrition and hydration reaching the skin's epidermis.

Moving on with more depressing stuff: you need to consider your age when you drink. For a twenty-year old, the alcohol leaves the body in about three hours. Unfortunately, a forty-year old will need a day and a half to cleanse the body of this aging menace. So, do the math, if you are older. **The Institute On Aging says a healthy sixty-five-year-old person can have seven drinks per week (no more than three at one time).** The key word here is HEALTHY: no health issues and no medications.

Ok, ok, ok, I know you will probably still have one or two, now and then, so here are some things you can do to improve the deleterious effects SPIRITS can do:

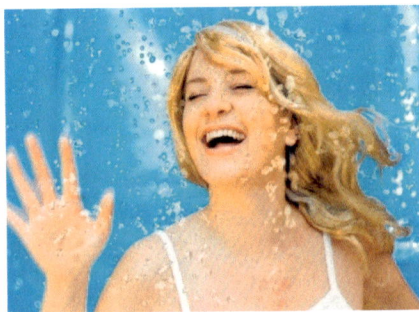

- Hydrate, hydrate, hydrate. Drink two to three pints of water before bed.
- Eat something before you drink and snack (non-sugary) while drinking to protect the lining of your stomach.
- Some suggest taking a spoon full of olive oil before endeavoring, to slow down absorption.

- Do not drink when on medications. Do I need to explain this?
- Do not drink if you have diabetes. It can cause drops and surges, and prevent meds from working.
- Do not drink if you are depressed or down. Call a friend or hotline first. Take a walk and pray.
- Exercise will help reduce the negative effects of alcohol consumption. Two and half hours of moderate exercise and activity per week is recommended. Regular exercise will reduce inflammation and damage to white matter in the brain. It will also reduce the dependence to alcohol by producing dopamine, the same feel-good hormone generated when drinking.
- Take n-acetyl cysteine before you drink to boost your glutathione levels and reduce toxic side effects.
- Restore a B deficiency (from drinking regularly) with a vitamin B complex.
- Take more vitamin C to replenish the deficiency that drinking causes. This vitamin is essential for the integrity of the skin.
- Add the nutritional supplement, milk thistle, to your regimen to protect your liver.
- Up your magnesium because it is depleted by alcohol consumption. It reduces inflammation and hangover symptoms.
- Add the antioxidant alpha lipoic acid to your regimen for skin renewal.
- Whiskey and rum have more congeners than vodka and gin. These little buggers are produced during fermentation and are responsible for hangovers! Some speculate, they could also do more damage to the skin. Skip the sugary mixers.
- Green nutritional food supplements tend to neutralize the effects of congeners.

- Tequila has less congeners and sugar, but skip the salt.
- Beer has antioxidants and less alcohol, drink slowly.
- White wine is high in sugar and has no none benefits. While red wine does cause flushing and redness, it does contain resveratrol, a powerful anti-aging antioxidant. It does help increase the HDL (good) cholesterol and increase hyaluronic acid in cells.
- There is a new type of wine called 'clean-crafted' produced by Scout & Cellar which is beyond organic. No dyes, no sugars, no added sulfites, no chemicals, no headaches! Learn more at *hellogorgeous.wine*.
- Obviously, eating a Clean Diet that is free of chemicals and toxins is priority if you are going to indulge occasionally.
- Juicing is a must to cleanse and detox. I love the *Big Book of Juices and Green Smoothies* by Cherie Calbom for great recipes.
- Love your skin more than you love drinking. Don't skip your nightly skin care regimen ever. Moisturize, moisturize, moisturize with a quality hydrating element like aloe vera. Do yourself a favor, and get my AM and PM Ultra Aloe Care moisturizers!

Believe me; this is for me, too, even though I didn't start indulging until I was around fifty. I discovered wine and fell in love. ☺

If you are going drink alcoholic beverages, then please incorporate all these helpful, healthy tips to prevent some of the damage they cause.

I hope you can see that if you want to live younger longer, you will have to drink less SPIRITS and drink them less often.

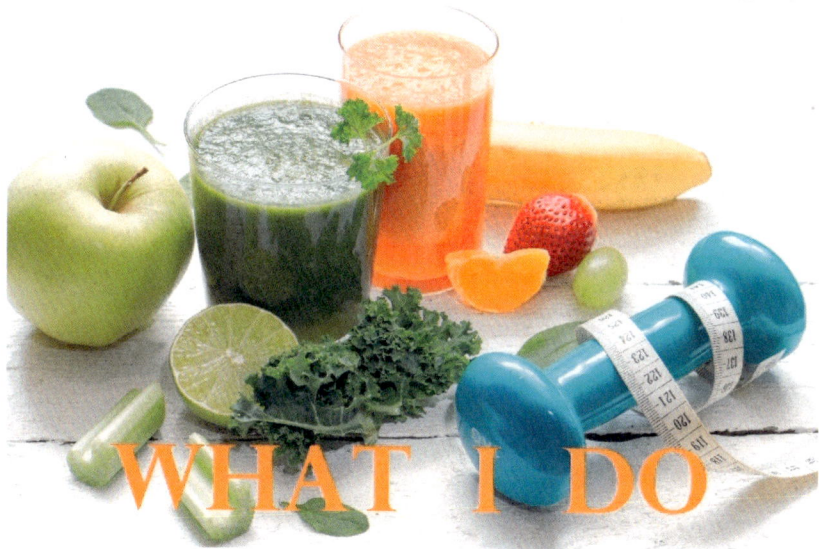

WHAT I DO

1. I never drink on an empty stomach.

2. I don't drink cocktails or cordials. My research recommends that if you do drink liquors, it's better to just drink shots or over ice. I have had a few shots of tequila!! ☺

3. I have found the most wonderful wine that gives no headaches, really! It is organic, non-GMO, no added sulfites or red dyes like mega-purple, no added sugar, and no added chemicals like ferrocyanide, copper sulfate, or ammonium phosphate found in most wine. Did you know that some wines have added the same amount of sugar that is found in a donut? Just think, if you have three glasses of wine, you have just consumed three donuts is some cases! For more information check out *hellogorgeous.wine*.

4. I only drink up to three glasses of wine at special events or parties.

5. I add ice to the second glass of wine if I know it's going to be a long night. Don't hate me wine people.

6. I drink at least two pints of filtered or spring water before I go to bed.

7. I take extra vitamin C, glutathione, and add 'green concentrate' to my breakfast smoothie.

8. I take a collagen booster supplement with hyaluronic acid.

9. Juicing and smoothies are part of my regular diet at least five times a week.

10. I do buy organic and follow the Dirty Dozen and Clean Fifteen recommendations.

11. I never, never, never go to bed without cleaning my face and putting on all my Hello Gorgeous anti-aging serums and moisturizer!

12. I use the HG dry skin line which includes hyaluronic acid, evening primrose, rose hips, sodium PCA, jojoba, and squalane. For more information go to *hellogorgeous.com*.

13. Finally, I try to do some form of exercising every day. Stretching, walking, bedroom workouts, dancing, or yoga. I think I will soon get an elliptical to use along with working out on my full body vibration machine!

Chapter 21

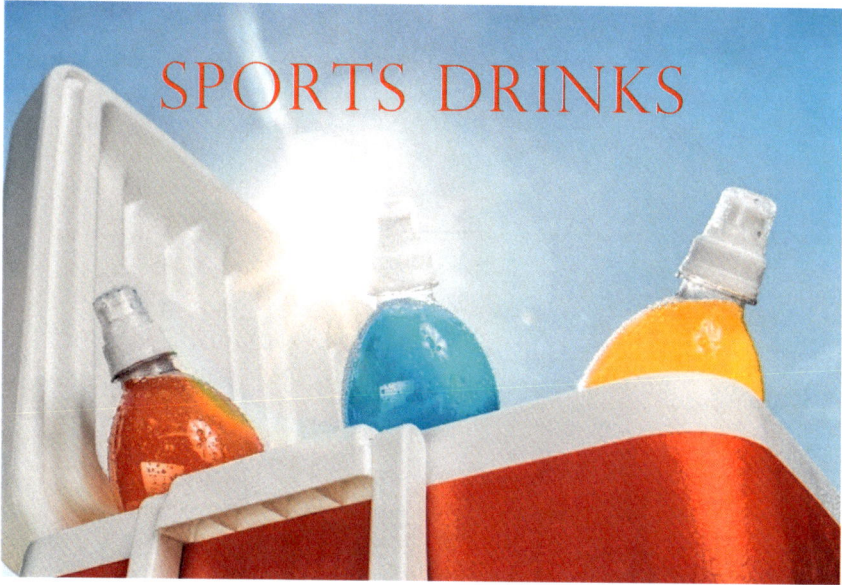

SPORTS DRINKS

It's hard to believe that SPORTS DRINKS and energy drinks have been on the scene around twenty-five years and is a twenty-five-billion-dollar industry. Today, they are the fastest growing beverage market as consumers believe them to be healthier than SODAS due to their association with sports and physical activity. The marketing gurus create brilliant advertisements promoting SPORTS DRINKS as a healthy way to re-hydrate, replenish electrolytes, and increase energy. **Is this true?**

I can visualize the mad scientists slaving over their blue and red concoctions of 400 mg of caffeine (equivalent to five cups of coffee) and 20g of SUGAR (five teaspoons of sugar), while throwing in a few exotic artificial dyes to make them more attractive on the shelf, and finishing with enough preservatives to make them last a decade or two.

I'm going to expose the dangers of SUGAR and its fake energy coming up. In this chapter let me help you see why true energy does not come from SPORTS DRINKS or energy drinks and how this deceptive advertising can be **deadly.**

The fuel for energy stored in your liver and muscle cells is called glycogen. Glycogen is basically the excess amount of glucose consumed from your diet that was not used for immediate energy. The average person stores enough glycogen for about ninety minutes of exercise.

Perhaps you have heard of carbohydrate loading, also known as, carb-loading or carbo-loading. Endurance athletes are encouraged to load up on carbs the week before an event to increase their amount of glycogen. They are not encouraged to load up on candy bars and sugary drinks; but grains, legumes, fruits and vegetables along with low-fat proteins. **Carb-loading does not mean gorging on pasta either.**

The combination of less training and a little extra carb-loading stores enough glycogen (usually a few extra pounds) which is easily converted to energy on the day of the big race for marathoners, bicyclists, and swimmers.

In order to convert the sugar from SPORTS DRINKS into glycogen, the body needs help from B vitamins, zinc, and manganese. Without these key nutrients (which are lacking from the fast-food diets of today,) insulin receptors are inhibited and AGEs (advanced glycation end-products) are produced. AGEs are basically free radicals that damage the cells in arteries, joints, eyes, and SKIN. (More information on AGEs is in SMOKED MEATS.)

AGEs produce oxidative stress on protein cell receptors forming cross-linking disrupting cellular structure and function. **SPORTS DRINKS (despite a few added vitamins) accelerate the aging process throughout the body as well as wrinkles in the SKIN.** They do nothing to enhance the athletic performance. Exercising causes enough free radical damage and SPORTS DRINKS just add more fuel to the flame.

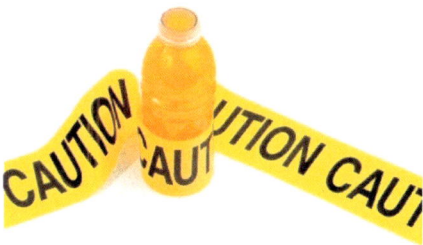

As for energy, the caffeine and herbal stimulates (usually guarana) in SPORTS DRINKS cause increased heart rate, high blood pressure, anxiety, and insomnia. The World Health Organization warns SPORTS DRINKS "may pose danger to public health." Dr. John Higgins, a sports cardiologist at the University of Texas Health Science Center in Houston, says that "energy drinks not only have been shown to raise stress levels, increase heart rate, and increase blood pressure; they've also been shown to make the blood a little bit thicker."

He explains these effects on the cardiovascular system are probably due to the interaction of caffeine and the other ingredients in these energy drinks like taurine. Taurine is an amino acid which affects the levels of water and minerals in the blood. **Toxicology reports from cardiac arrest patients drinking SPORTS DRINKS report high levels of caffeine and taurine.** In one case of a twenty-eight-year-old, "His arteries of the heart were completely locked up," says Dr. Higgins.

The phosphates and sodium citrate, used as preservatives in SPORTS DRINKS, makes an acidic environment that stresses the immune system. To compensate, the body tries to restore tissue alkalinity by tapping into calcium and magnesium reserves in the bones, leading eventually to osteoporosis.

Then there are BVOs (brominated vegetable oil) that keep flavors dispersed. Numerous studies, according to *WebMD*, show a build-up in the body can cause headaches, fatigue, loss of muscle coordination, loss of memory, and serious skin conditions. Artificial dyes can cause DNA, liver and brain damage as published in studies on *PubMed.gov*.

SPORTS DRINKS and energy drinks are not the answer to boost your health and hydration during physical activity. Even water with electrolytes is usually made of processed salt which just increases your sodium load. Be aware of 'sugar-free' versions as well, because the artificial SWEETENERS add even more toxins.

So, what do you do? Drink natural spring water! For electrolytes, add sea salt or Himalayan salt to natural spring water. Coconut water contains the highest sources of electrolytes on the planet for those profusely sweating work-outs and sports activities.

To enhance your athletic performance, eat real food and drink real water that hasn't been GMO'd, hydrogenated, brominated, dyed, electrolyzed, enhanced, or created. Buy yourself a few beverage containers in your favorite colors, fill with spring water, and quench your thirst naturally. If you want to live younger longer, SPORTS DRINKS should not be on your shopping list.

Natural hydration keeps your blood, your heart, your brain, and your skin young!

WHAT I DO

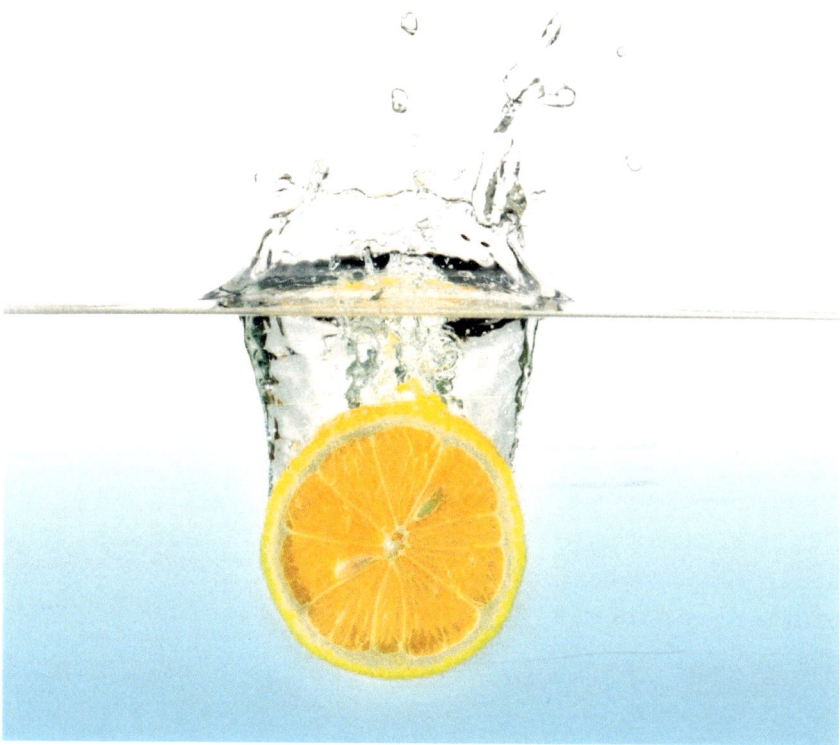

1. I drink Fiji water, natural spring water, and Berkey filtered water.

2. I add lemon juice to water, smoothies, juicing, and tea.

3. I don't drink SPORTS DRINKS, energy drinks, or water with electrolytes.

4. I bring a small container of Himalayan salt with me at all times.

5. I make 'spa water' for home and work which is water with sliced fresh fruit: oranges, lemons, cucumbers, berries, mint, apples, pineapple, etc.

6. My diet includes plenty of fresh fruits, vegetables, protein, and good fats.

7. I take B complex (key in converting food into fuel), coenzyme Q10 (cellular energy), magnesium and zinc (muscle recovery and zinc is great for skin), omega 3 EPA and DHA (reduces inflammation), and amino acids (organic plant protein powders to drink within 30 minutes after workout or physical activities.)

Chapter 22

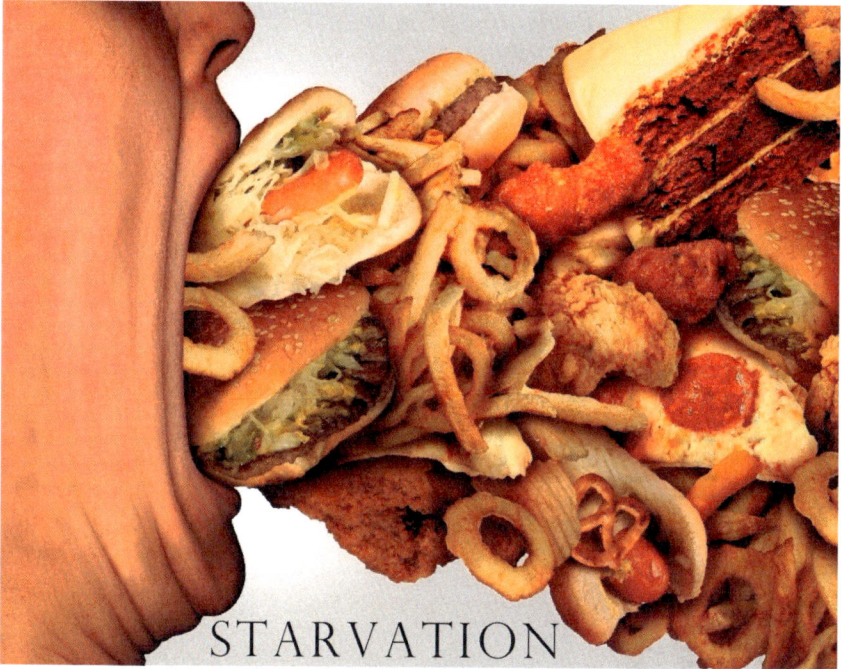

STARVATION

Most people in America do not look like they are starving since **they are eating sixty to seventy tons of food during a lifetime**, but they are. In fact, according to the World Food Clock, eleven million pounds of food are consumed worldwide every minute of every day. So, how is STARVATION a factor in aging and longevity?

The human body is made up of fifty trillion cells that produce billions of chemical reactions every second of every day. Did you know your heart beats one hundred thousand times a day? Did you know that every month you completely regenerate your outer layer of skin? Did you know every three months you rebuild and replace your blood supply and every ten years, adults rebuild every bone in their body?

Most Americans are not getting the nutrition they need to produce the billions of chemical reactions that renew and rebuild every part of our bodies, inside and out. **Dr. Libby Weaver says that "we are living too short and dying too long."** If your diet is not made up of fresh ingredients (not from a box, package or can), your cells are STARVING. Given the right ingredients for optimum cellular nutrition, your body can keep you young and healthy for a long time.

Have you heard of Eating Clean? Basically, it is choosing to eliminate all processed food and extra additives from your diet by eating whole, unrefined foods. Whole foods provide an adequate amount of essential nutrients and minerals.

By eating a wide variety of whole foods, you will ensure any nutritional void will be filled. You could pop a lot of vitamins, but whole foods actually provide more readily absorbed vitamins and minerals. **You can prevent cellular STARVATION.**

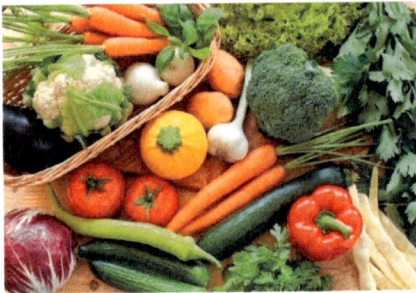

How many times must I say, you have to eat fresh fruits and vegetables? Each year the Environmental Working Group (EWG) puts out a guide to pesticides retained in produce called 'The Dirty Dozen' and 'The Clean Fifteen.' It helps you know which vegetables and fruits that you should buy organic because of too much contamination.

The Dirty Dozen usually looks something like this: strawberries, spinach, nectarines, apples, peaches, pears, cherries, grapes, celery, tomatoes, sweet bell peppers, and potatoes. If you buy these, buy organic. The scores for cucumbers, cherry tomatoes, lettuce, snap peas, and blueberries are not usually far behind.

The Clean Fifteen (meaning the least amount of pesticides measured) are usually sweet corn, avocados, pineapples, cabbage, onions, sweet peas (frozen), papayas, asparagus, mangos, eggplant, honeydew melon, kiwi, cantaloupe, cauliflower, and grapefruit.

Some sweet corn, papaya and summer squash sold in America are made with genetically modified seeds (GMO) which means the pesticide is built into the seed. They don't necessarily show up on the list. That is why you should buy non-GMO fruits and vegetables and check the EWG website each year.

Non-GMO might even be more important than organic because the percentage of Americans with three or more chronic illnesses has jumped from seven percent to thirteen percent in just nine years after the introduction of genetically modified organisms. Allergies, autism, reproductive disorders, digestive problems, and others are also skyrocketing.

- Eating Clean means eating grass-fed beef, lamb, game, poultry, eggs, and wild-caught fish.

- Eating Clean means eating organic and non-GMO grains, legumes, fruits and vegetables.

- Eating Clean means drinking filtered water or spring water.

- Eating Clean will provide the cellular nutrition you need without clogging the works with deadly chemicals that cancel the nutritional benefits.

It's also important to know the role fat plays in your health. There are good fats (naturally-made) and bad fats (man-altered). Eating

Clean means eating good fats, as well. Bad fats will cause cellular STARVATION and diseases from inflammation.

A word about **GOOD FAT**: Good fats produce hormones, good digestion, energy, and optimal mental function which are important for seniors. It is the preferred fuel of the body. Did you know that your brain is sixty to sixty-five percent saturated fat? Saturated fats are not the demons they were once thought to be.

All-natural fats are good for you no matter whether they are saturated, monounsaturated, or polyunsaturated. You need fat to make healthy cell walls which are flexible and permeable. Lamb and beef fat contain stearic acid which lowers cholesterol, provides vitamin E, and has no free-radicals when heated.

Even lard has antimicrobials, vitamins A, D, and K2. Butterfat has anti-cancer CLA and vitamins A, D, and K. Coconut oil has antiviral capabilities and balances HDL/LDL ratios. In fact, all-natural saturated fats raise HDL (good cholesterol) and increase bone mineral density. **Saturated fats are not the kiss of death as once supposed, but rather the low-fat diet is!**

By now you have probably heard of a hot new name for certain saturated fats called MCT oil. This refers to medium-chain fatty acids and compared to longer-chain fats (more carbon bonds), MCTs are more easily digested and absorbed. Since they are sent directly to the liver, they increase metabolism and are utilized for energy over glucose.

While there are MCTs in coconut oil and grass-fed butter, cheese, and whole milk, MCT oil is only short-chain fatty acid. More information on how MCT oil improves cognition, reduces cardiovascular disease, and promotes weight loss is found the book *The Bulletproof Diet* and *Draxe.com.*

Other good fats are monounsaturated fats like olive oil which contains oleic acid which reduces inflammation. It also contains antioxidants vitamins E and K, and lowers the risk of stroke and heart disease. Other good fats come from avocados, walnuts, almonds, pistachios, seeds, fish, and eggs. Good fat is not your enemy. **Good fat does not make you fat, sugar does**! So please remove the word 'low-fat' from your vocabulary.

A word about **BAD FAT**: Bad fat, also known as trans-fat, is your enemy. Early in the twentieth century, food companies learned how to extend the life of oils by adding hydrogen atoms to the carbon chain making them turn into solid (margarine and vegetable shortening.)

'Partially hydrogenated oil' is now a clever marketing concept (not a healthy alternative), as scientists discovered a new way of chemically altering oils for frying and packaged foods. Trans-fats, aka bad fats, increase LDL (bad cholesterol) and inflammation which is linked to diabetes, stroke, heart disease, etc.

Consuming only two percent of your calories from trans-fats increases the risk of heart disease by twenty-three percent. This man-made fat has no known health benefits.

Eliminate hydrogenated and partially hydrogenated oils like soy, corn, canola, cotton seed, sunflower, and safflower. Eliminate margarine and fake spreads. Read labels before buying anything to look for this FAKE FOOD.

Use coconut oil, olive oil, and real butter.

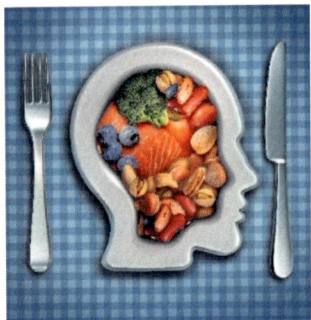

Your BRAIN is STARVING too! The brain is only two percent of your body weight (about three lbs.) but uses twenty-five percent of the calories you consume. Obviously, the brain is the most complex organ in the body, but even though it is relatively small it is the most metabolically active as well.

Known as the 'hungry organ' the body gives it the first bite of every food it consumes which is why your diet is so important.

- Protein is the building block for all cells, maintaining and repairing all bodily systems and is responsible for a lifetime of growth and development. Neurotransmission (chemical messaging) is dependent on amino acids which are the raw material of protein. Meat, fish, poultry, and some dairy are best sources (when organic, free-range, grass-fed and deep-water sourced).

- Fat is necessary for all the processes of the brain. The body can make most of the fatty acids it needs, except omega-3 and 6, also known as essential fatty acids. Cold-water oily fish such as sardines, salmon, mackerel, pilchards, herring, trout, and tuna are good choices to add to your diet. Flaxseed oil and fish oil supplements are other good sources. Eggs contain lecithin necessary for brain signaling and organ meats contain important phospholipids. Fat from avocados, nuts, seeds, and olive oil are important as well.

- Carbohydrates (grains and legumes) in their natural, unrefined, unprocessed state release their sugar content slowly into the bloodstream and onto the brain. Though not as important as fat and protein, are needed for optimum brain function.

- Vegetables, fruits and spices are now known to have regenerative effects on the brain. Turmeric and rosemary are the stars in the spice world. Sulforaphanes and Vitamin K from cruciferous vegetables (especially broccoli sprouts) and lutein and zeaxanthin from spinach and kale repair, protect, and regenerate brain cells. Blueberries and pomegranate are the best fruits.

Unfortunately, the Standard American Diet is SAD because it is mostly dead food laden with sugars, table salt, hydrogenated oils, over-processed grains, and chemicals that our cells do not recognize as food to fuel cellular energy to regenerate and rebuild. No wonder we cannot live out our lives with good health and happiness. Our cells are STARVING.

Food can be either constructive or destructive. Did you know that many signs of aging are the beginning of chronic disease? If you want to look younger and live healthier longer, you must change the way you eat and what you eat. Review the anti-inflammatory diet in SMOLDERING KILLER.

Remember to friend my FB page *Color Me Thin*, for healthy eating strategies and others like David Wolfe and *Goodful*. Also, more great info is on my new website *WholelifeNutrition.me*.

It's time to get back into the kitchen and cook healthy, nutritious meals.

End STARVATION by feeding your cells properly!

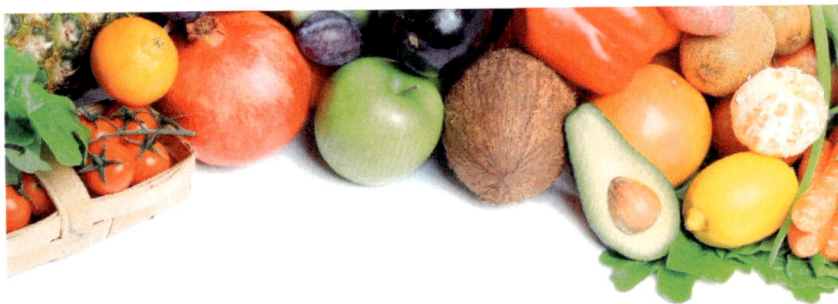

WHAT I DO

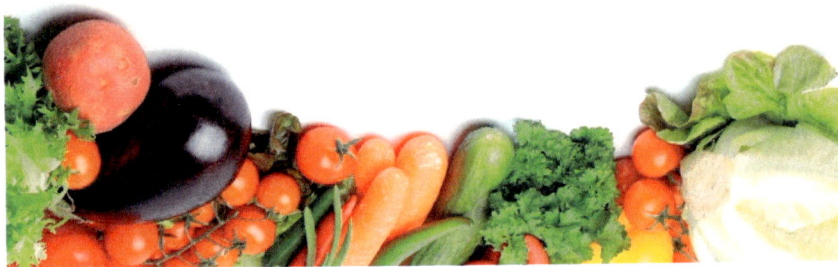

1. I start each day with a glass of lemon water or vinegar water to help maintain an alkaline state.

2. While I love to make veggie and cheese frittatas on the weekends, I have protein and collagen shakes or smoothies for breakfast with blueberries, nuts or avocado, lemon, greens, and almond milk. Lots of great recipes are out there which include nut butters as well.

3. I drink loads of green tea. I also love oolong for energy, white tea, and ginger and turmeric herbal teas as well.

4. I eat nuts and seeds between meals as well as, berries, grapefruit, and avocado.

5. I love to juice. It's a great way to skip a meal, but only juice if you can drink it immediately. Here are three great recipes I learned about at nutrition school:

Green Vitality:
1 cup of spinach, 2 celery stalks, ½ peeled cucumber,
1 green apple cored, 1 handful of parsley, and
juice from half a lemon and a lime.

Red Energy:
1 beet root, 2 carrots, 2 celery stalks,
and 2 plum tomatoes.

Orange Immunity:
1/2 a cored and peeled pineapple, 1 peeled orange,
2 large carrots, ½ inch peeled ginger root,
and ½ peeled lemon.

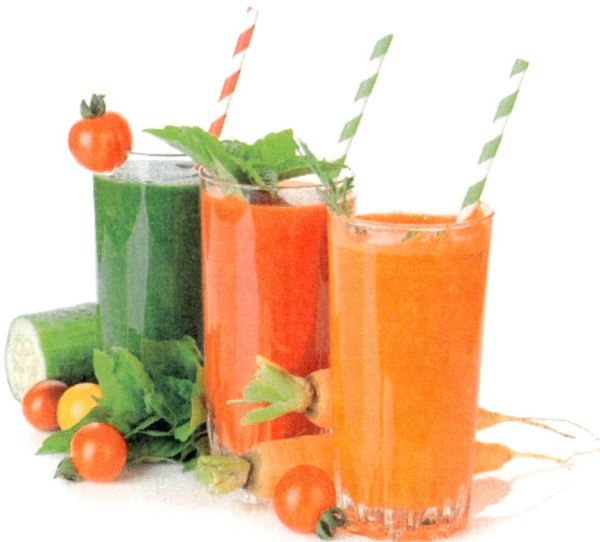

6. I eat the Color Me Thin way! It's a simple premise I have
    created to keep the body more alkaline where disease cannot
    flourish. Simply eat ¾ of your plate with colorful fruits and
    vegetables and ¼ of your plate is left for animal or fish protein
    and/or whole grains/legumes.

7. The Color Me Thin way limits dairy and avoids all white stuff like flour, sugar, potatoes, white rice, and pasta. The Color Me Thin way cooks with good fats like butter, coconut oil and olive oil. When you look at your plate and all you see is brown, white and beige, to be blunt, you are getting fat and sick. ☺

8. I eat one-third of my diet raw (salads, fruits, nuts, and veggies.) Lycopene from tomatoes, red bell peppers, watermelon, red cabbage, guava, mango, and grapefruit is a great skin protecting anti-oxidant and boosts the level of procollagen in the skin.

9. Fats are important. I avoid anything that says Fat-Free or contains hydrogenated oils. I drizzle olive oil and cook with coconut oil.

10. I cook with loads of spices because they help with inflammation: garlic, ginger, turmeric, curry powder, chili powder, basil, rosemary, thyme, and cinnamon.

11. My favorite dessert is dark chocolate seventy-two percent or higher.

12. I do cook some grains like wild rice or brown rice, barley, amaranth, or quinoa. But I keep them to small proportions more like a condiment or plating accent when serving animal or fish protein.

13. I only cook gluten-free pasta no more than once a month. I love to use spaghetti squash instead.

14. I don't eat anything that says Sugar-Free or has more than 4g of sugar on the label.

15. I take probiotics and eat real fermented pickles and sauerkraut.

16. Even though I eat an organic, clean diet, I take a few anti-oxidants to squelch the free radical damage that just naturally

occurs each day. As we age, we need all the help we can get. Resveratrol, Astaxanthin, vitamin C, coenzyme Q10, and L-glutathione are my favorites.

17. When organic is not available, wash your vegetables with a little SLS-free soap in a sink full of water to rinse off pesticide residue. You can also spray a mixture of hydrogen peroxide (one teaspoon) in eight ounces of water on them.

Chapter 23

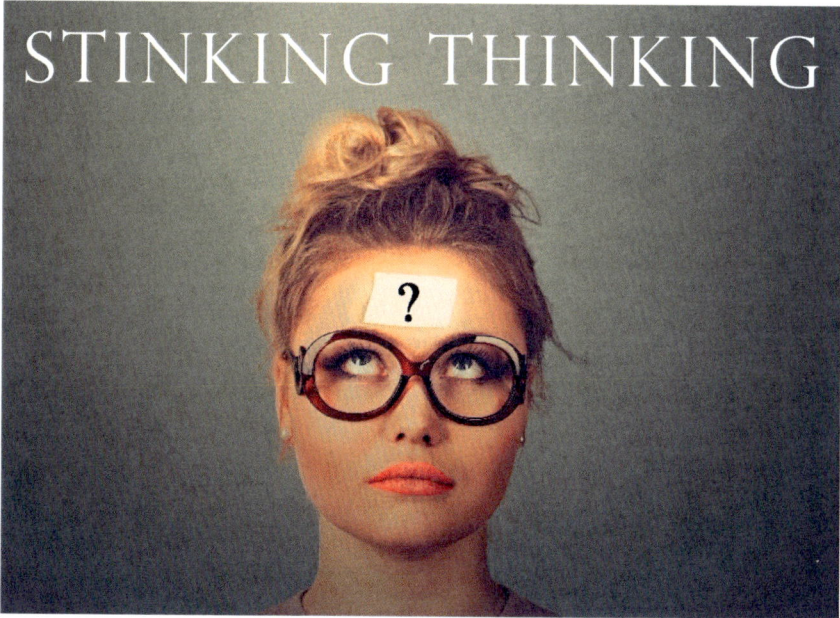

STINKING THINKING

What is STINKING THINKING? Did you know that if you think you are old, then you will be? Did you know that your feelings become your chemistry? **Science now verifies that your genes make you vulnerable, but your thoughts and behavior trigger them.**

Dr. Deepak Chopra says your emotions are directly linked to your biology. He explains a new science, called Epigenetics, is emerging and finds that even though the sequence of your DNA is fixed, how you turn on your genes or turn them off depends on the quality of your awareness.

Your thoughts, your feelings, emotions, speech, diet, language, relationships, sleep, etc. actually influence the way your genes are regulated. He goes on to say that only five percent of your genes are penetrant (cannot be changed like Down syndrome), but ninety-five percent are controlled by you. You can turn on the good ones and turn off the bad ones just by your lifestyle choices.

It is estimated that the average person has over seventy thousand thoughts per day. What are your thoughts saying? Are they positive and uplifting? Or are they negative and self-defeating?

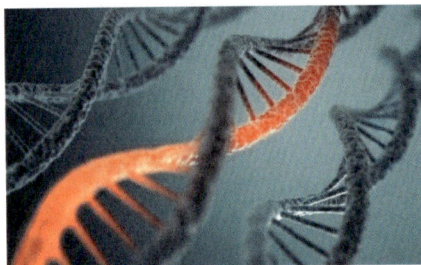

Scientists who study neuroplasticity believe that some of the most powerful neurotransmitters in your brain are your emotions. Neuroplasticity means that the brain physically changes with every thought and experience. It's amazing that the one hundred billion neurons in your brain depend on the state of your consciousness or awareness.

- Dr. Caroline Leaf tells us that a thought makes a permanent neuro pathway in your brain if you focus on it seven or more times. You must realize that your thoughts become reality. You are in control of creating brain matter and functions just by what you think and believe.

- Ralph Waldo Emerson said: "You are what you think you are, all day long."

- James Allen said: "You are today where your thoughts have brought you. You will be tomorrow where your thoughts take you."

- Keith D. Harrell said: "If you can imagine it, you can achieve it. If you dream it, you can become it."

- The *Bible* says, "As a man thinketh in his heart, so is he." Proverbs: 23:7.

Is your mind filled with love, joy, happiness, peace, contentment, kindness, forgiveness, and self-acceptance? Do you think you are a happy, positive person? Is your mind full of negative self-talk, wounds, unforgiveness, jealousy, or shame?

Cheryl Grey, a professional counselor, says that self-image is based on the relationship you have with yourself and the relationship is based on what you believe about yourself and what you believe about yourself is based on thoughts. According to her research, thoughts come from two sources:

1) What others have said about you that you have come into agreement with.

2) Your interpretation of the events and circumstances of your life.

So, what have others said about you? If those words were not positive, encouraging, helpful, and kind, don't let them take up residence in your brain. How have you interpreted the things that have happened to you? **Have they made you better or bitter?**

I don't think I know anyone who has led a charmed life. No one I know is perfect. No one I know is free of wounds and injustice. But I do know a lot of people (including me) who know how to turn challenges into opportunities and who have left their old baggage at the station of regret to board the train to a new now.

The unpleasant circumstances or events in your life are not a sign that you are not worthy or special. You were created to bring a special kind of light into this world. You were designed to shine! What is your specialty? Don't let the unkind words or deeds of the past put out your light, because you will not be the real, authentic, awesome you.

I hope that you can see that STINKING THINKING can ruin your chances for a successful, happy, healthy life.

According to Dr. Leaf's research, even science has now determined that humans were created to love and not hate, to think good and positive thoughts. When you do, the correct chemicals are produced by the hypothalamus and you are happy and healthy.

Toxic thoughts are unnatural to you and produce cortisol, the stress hormone also known as the death hormone. They will take you on an unhealthy route to sickness and disease. Your body must love and be happy to function optimally. And it all starts with what you are thinking!

- Have an inner circle of uplifting and positive friends
- Do something kind for someone every day
- Find three things to be grateful for every day
- Do something positive for yourself each day
- Close your eyes when you hear negative self-talk and put those words in a box and bury them
- Dr. Daniel Amen, psychiatrist, says to talk back to your feelings. When you are feeling sad, mad, nervous, out of control, etc. just write the feelings down on a piece of paper and talk back to them. (He says it will save you years of therapy).
- Determine what your signature strengths are and commit to using them in new ways each week (learn more at *authentichappiness.com*)

- Renew your mind with books and classes that will improve your state of being (The *Bible* is always my number one go-to book)

- Set aside time for relationships, playtime, movement, good sleep, good food, and prayerful meditation

- Believe that you are Beautiful

- Realize that the best time in your life is right NOW

- Understand that all things do work together for your good (Romans 8:28).

What you believe is critical to your health and longevity. Thirty-five percent of placebo participants get well because they believe they are getting the cure.

Scientists can determine how long you will live by asking you two questions:

1) How long do you think you will live?

2) How many fruits and vegetables do you eat?

If you think you are running out of time, your blood will become thick and sluggish, you will have a heart attack and you **WILL** run out of time, explains Dr. Chopra.

If you want to live younger longer, you must abandon STINKING THINKING in all areas of your life!

WHAT I DO

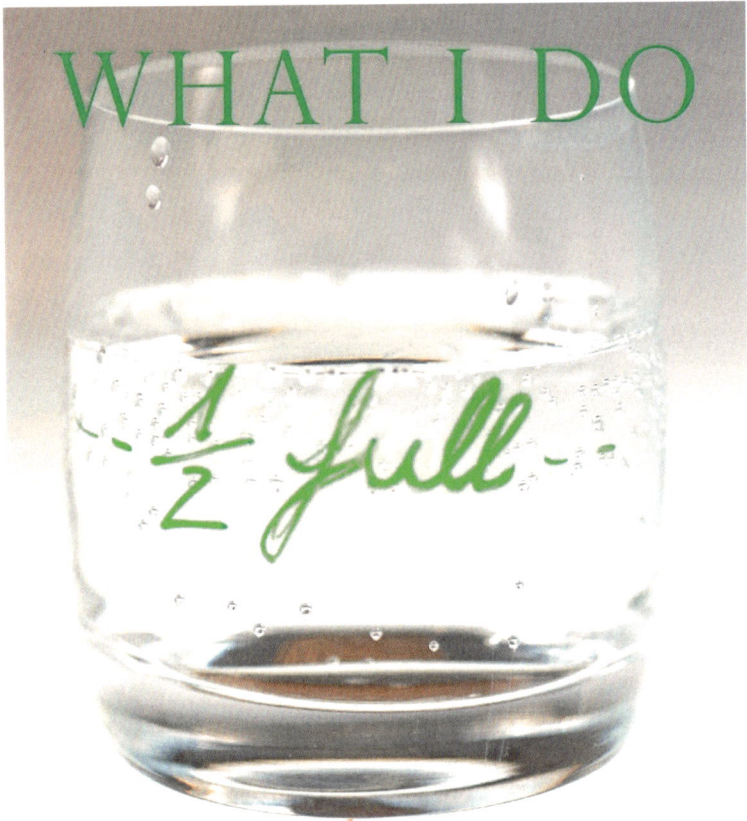

1. I get up every day and put makeup on after my AM facial regimen. It may only be mascara and lipstick if I am staying at home for the day, but it makes me feel good when I look in the mirror!

2. I love to laugh and watch funny sitcoms or movies. One of our health instructors told us to laugh five times a day.

3. I try to get rid of unforgiveness as fast as I get it.

4. I get rid of negative self-thoughts as fast as I get them.

5. I always think the glass is half full, not half empty.

6. I try to see that life is full of teachable moments and see how everything works together for my good.

7. I get together with girlfriends as often as I can.

8. I give thanks anytime something comes to mind.

9. I have been studying Spanish for two years to keep my brain in a learning mode and to speak this beautiful language. My grandchildren are bilingual too!!

10. I make time to do some form of exercise every day. It's my: me-time!

11. I read books that teach me something new to add to my knowledge.

12. I smile a lot. It keeps my face young.

13. I love to find things my husband and I can do. Whether it's a concert, movie, vacation, dinner, festival, etc. I like to make time to smell the roses.

14. I believe that all things are possible all the time.

Chapter 24

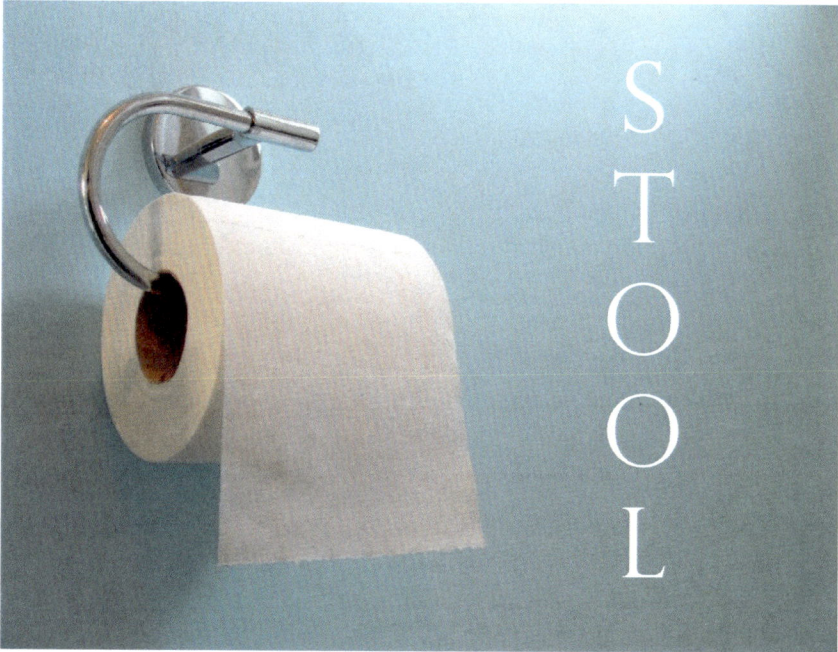

I apologize for bringing this topic up, **but your STOOL may be trying to tell you something.** I'm going to make this a short one, but eliminating fecal matter properly is important to living a long heathy life. ☺

Normal bowel movements vary from person to person. It could be one to three times a day or three or four times per week. Passing gas is normal (fourteen times per day) so you won't blow up like a balloon. It usually goes undetected. Proper bowel transit time is between twelve to twenty-four hours to allow enough time to absorb all the water and nutrients. Bowel transit time is faster however, if you eat mostly insoluble fiber.

Please check out the 'Bristol Stool Chart' to determine what kind of STOOL you have. The size, texture, shape, and color are important and this chart is a great guide. Ideally, you should be type 3, 4, or 5 with type 4 being the 'Holy Grail' of STOOL.

Bristol Stool Chart

Type 1	●● ●●	Separate hard lumps, like nuts (hard to pass)
Type 2		Sausage-shaped but lumpy
Type 3		Like a sausage but with cracks on its surface
Type 4		Like a sausage or snake, smooth and soft
Type 5		Soft blobs with clear-cut edges (passed easily)
Type 6		Fluffy pieces with ragged edges, a mushy stool
Type 7		Watery, no solid pieces. **Entirely Liquid**

You may need to bulk up on fiber if you are type 6 or 7. You may need to consider lactose intolerance, adverse reaction to artificial sweeteners or fructose, or you may be gluten intolerant if type 6 or 7. This could imply diseases like celiac, Crohn's, ulcerative colitis, IBS, hypothyroidism, or gastrointestinal infection. If you have type 1 or 2, this could lead to fecal impaction which can be a serious medical condition.

People sixty-five and older are at higher risk of constipation and should use laxatives only as a last resort. Diabetes, IBS, hypothyroidism, and other health issues can cause constipation. Eating more fruits and vegetables, exercise, and drinking more water is your first line of defense.

- **SOLUBLE FIBER** slows digestion because it absorbs water and turns to gel in the intestines and does not get fully digested. Sources soluble fiber include grains like oat bran and barley; legumes like beans, lentils, and peas; vegetables like Brussel sprouts, turnips, sweet potatoes, and carrots; fruits like grapefruit, oranges, apricots, mangoes, and bananas; and flaxseed.

Those of you with types 6 and 7 STOOL, need to add more soluble fiber to their diet. This helps alleviate diarrhea since it attracts water to remove excess fluid.

- **INSOLUBLE FIBER** does not absorb water; it pulls water into the colon, and passes through close to its original form. It helps prevent constipation since it acts like a sweeper, pushing waste along.

While most insoluble fiber comes from the bran layers of cereal grains (whole grains) and brown rice other sources are dark, leafy vegetables, cabbage, zucchini, broccoli, root vegetables, okra, corn, grapes, berries, nuts, and seeds.

STOOL types 1 and 2 will benefit highly with more insoluble fiber and eliminating white bread, refined cereals, and white rice.

Proper elimination reduces toxic build-up in your skin. Need I say more? **If you want to have beautiful skin, you will need to poop properly. Ok, I said it.**

Your STOOL is important to your health and longevity. Do your research and learn more about this 'S' Word. Consider the medications you are taking and possible side effects. Eat more organic, whole foods like fresh vegetables for fiber, not grains.

You may need to avoid gluten and lactose. Avoid artificial sweeteners and excess sugar. Squat instead of sit! Avoid stress!

Get STOOL smart. It will help you live a longer, younger, healthier life

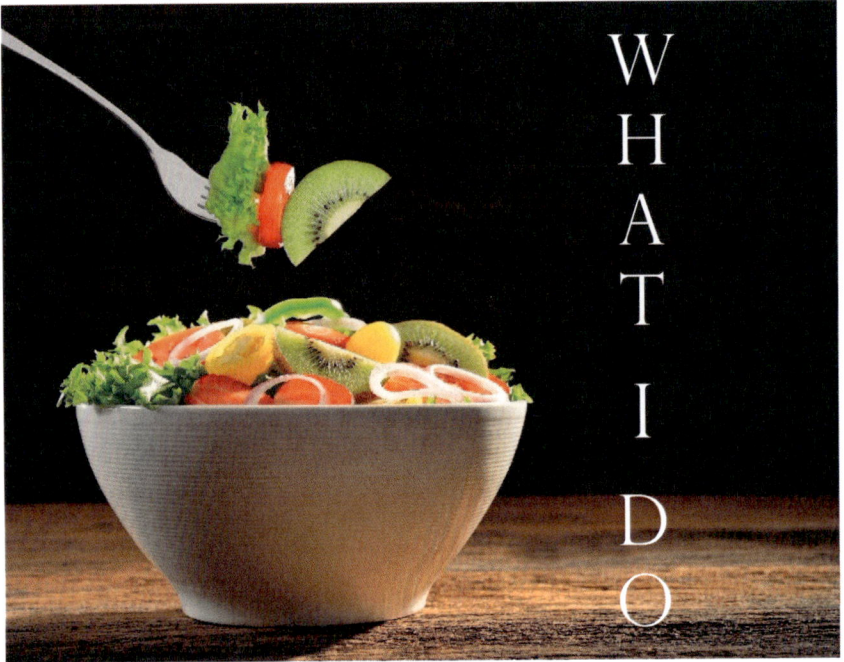

W
H
A
T

I

D
O

1. By now you should know I eat loads of fresh fruits and vegetables.

2. I eat only whole gluten-free grains, but sparingly as condiments to my meals.

3. I avoid gluten, lactose, and artificial sweeteners as they are triggers to diarrhea.

4. I use lactose-free milk products sparingly.

5. I eat fermented vegetables for the pro-biotics.

6. I take pro-biotics.

7. If I get a blemish on my face, I check out our facial chart to see where the problem is coming from.

Chapter 25

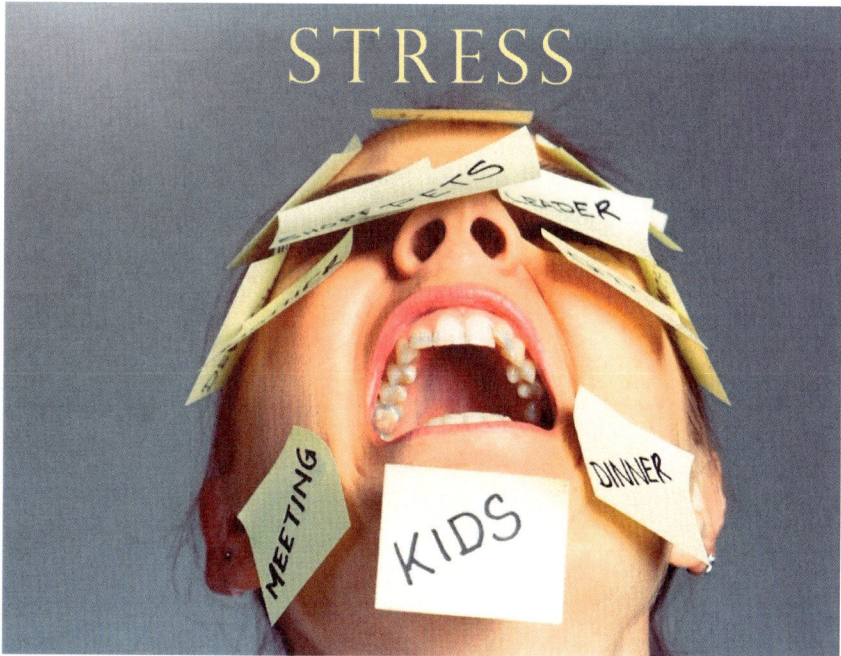

STRESS is a normal reaction to exciting events. Unfortunately, though, because it is a hardwired survival technique built into your body as a means of protection; **it does not know the difference between your boss yelling at you or a bear chasing you.**

So, STRESS is good when you are in danger, your adrenals secrete glucocorticoid hormones like cortisol and epinephrine (adrenalin) equipping you with emergency fuel and energy.

The extended release of STRESS hormones has an adverse effect on your body and will affect your health and longevity.
Even though your body reacts within milliseconds to stress, it takes the immune system much longer to respond. That means, sudden or short-lived stressful situations do not affect the immune system, but chronic on-going stress keeps cortisol pumping through your

veins and cortisol prevents the immune cells from responding to foreign invaders like viruses, infections, and cancer cells.

- Constant STRESS triggers anger, depression, sleep issues, high blood pressure and heart rate, higher cholesterol, heart attack risk, fat storage, hunger pains, lower immune function, acid reflux, stomach cramps, nausea, low libido, low sperm count, irregular cycles, low bone density, muscle pains, cystic breasts, back pain, and knee weakness according *WebMD*.

- High cortisol levels trigger oil production and inflammation. This creates an environment that spurs the growth of bacteria leading to clogged and enlarged pores and acne.

- Chronic inflammation leads to visible FACIAL signs of aging like fine lines and wrinkles, fragility and laxity due to collagen destruction and tissue atrophy. Facial STRESS also includes dark circles and excessive pigmentation. Not to mention what harsh facial expressions can do!

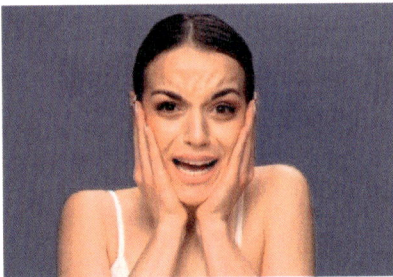

Constant STRESS rewires the circuitry of your brain. STRESS chemicals shrink your memories temporarily, and you cannot use them until these bad boys have subsided allowing the memories to plump back up again, according to Dr. Carolyn Leaf of Dallas, Texas. **She warns that if you don't get STRESS under control, over time these chemicals will literally attack the memories and eat them.**

- According to Karen Young at *HeySigmund.com*, exposure to toxic STRESS during your adulthood will intensify the aging process and affect memory, cognition, and emotions.

The National Institute On Mental Health tells us that anxiety disorders are currently the most common mental illness in the U.S. Over forty million adults (eighteen percent of the population) are **currently being treated at a cost of forty-two billion dollars**, which is one third of our total U.S. medical costs.

Some of the most widely prescribed drugs are opioids (pain killers) along with anxiety (Xanax and Valium) medications. According to *WebMD*, a new U.S. study shows that even though thirty percent of fatal overdoses incudes this fatal combination, the number of people prescribed both has spiked.

The total list of side effects is too long to mention here, but is easily found on the internet. **You should know that if the STRESS doesn't kill you, the negative side effects of these medications can.** You are just trading one problem for another.

Dr. Nadia Kumentas of Toronto has a great article about the new studies of L-theanine, a potent amino acid that is found in tea. New evidence reveals that L-theanine is a natural substitute for anti-stress drugs working as a relaxing agent with no harmful side effects. Like prescription drugs it interacts with brain receptors and increases dopamine (the feel-good hormone), GABA, and glycine levels. According to Dr. Kumentas, by calming the nervous system, it reduces the perception of stress and increases alpha-waves which keep you alert but calm.

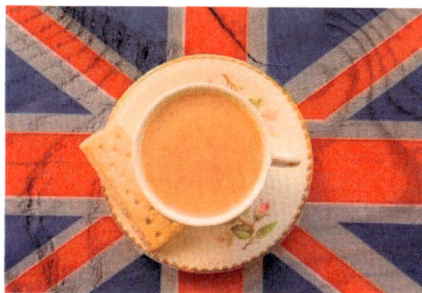

I never thought I would say this, but the British have been doing something right all these years. They take many 'time-outs' for tea and they do seem pretty calm (my husband is British). ☺

Black tea and Matcha green tea are the most potent, but Matcha green tea has the added bonus of more anti-oxidants! I sprinkle it into my green tea. That must be why I am so calm, cool, and collected.

Taking relaxing warm salt baths is a great way to relax and de-stress. Epsom salt comes from natural springs in England and has been recommended for decades to soothe aching muscles. It breaks down into magnesium and sulfate which induces relaxation. Dead Sea salts and Himalayan pink salt have more minerals and can even improve skin conditions, arthritis, and other health problems. I would avoid artificially colored and perfumed salts.

Make time for prayer and meditation. Practice calming activities like yoga, walking, or stretching. A short trip to a park or open space provides the same opportunity to relax. Cut back on carbs, sugar, and caffeine. Eat fresh whole foods. Instead of a 'coffee break' have a 'tea break.'

Obviously, STRESS is very aging and harmful to your health. You will have to reduce the tension in your life. That may mean taking some drastic measures like moving, changing jobs, setting boundaries with family members and friends, putting yourself 'first' for a change, etc.

Get serious about taking care of yourself, especially your skin. Don't let STRESS steal your joy and this time on earth.

What do hugs, hobbies, friendships, holidays, loving your job, sports, exercise, and eating more fruits and vegetables have in common? STRESS busters, of course.

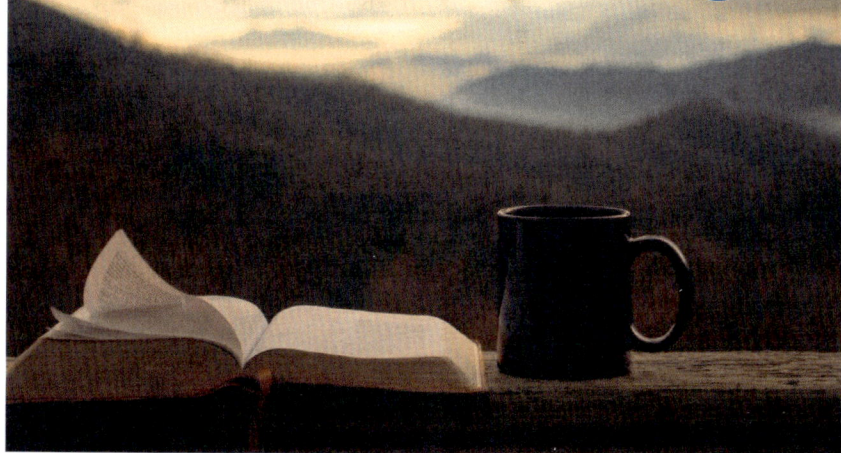

WHAT I DO

1. I love to sit outside in our outdoor living area with a cup of tea or glass of wine. I listen to the water fall, watch the birds, and just enjoy the view. We live on a golf course, so lots of green grass and blue sky to see.

2. I practice the 4 R's: Realize where STRESS is coming from. Do all you can do to Resolve it. Release it to God so He can align your future to Receive the answer.

3. I practice deep breathing techniques. **This is breathing with your tummy, not your chest**. Place your hand on your tummy and breathe in through your nose with your diaphragm counting to seven (your chest should not move). Then release the air through your mouth counting to seven. You can do this anytime. As you do this, you focus on your breath and nothing else. This is a type of meditation and a simplified version of the new movement called mindfulness. According to the magazine, *The Power of Mindfulness*, "There's been a surge in research over the past decade geared toward understanding how nonjudgmental awareness of thoughts,

feelings and sensations improves our well-being. Mindfulness inserts a pause into a behavioral cascade, helping to override emotional impulses." In my words: it reduces the production of the stress hormone, cortisol, and trains you to respond to events in a more calm manner. Just sit and breathe.

4. I only have one cup of coffee in the morning with a pinch of baking soda to neutralize the acidity. (OK, maybe two.)

5. I drink green tea (with Matcha) during the day, which has about a third of the caffeine of coffee. At night, though, I drink herbal teas or caffeine-free varieties. Curbing caffeine is a must if you are stressed, but as you have just learned tea is a de-stressor.

6. I love walnuts. Turns out they increase serotonin levels which is the hormone that creates calm and happiness.

7. I get at least eight hours of sleep every night.

8. I drink tea through-out the day.

9. I have a really deep tub for taking hot salt baths. I use Himalayan crystals or Epsom salt.

10. I never forget my HG skin care regimens no matter how I feel. As I have already mentioned, our skin care is aloe-based. Aloe vera is probably the best anti-inflammatory agent on the planet. It blocks harmful enzymes, MMPs (matrix metalloproteinases), which cause tissue damage and inhibits prostanoid production which produces swelling and pain. Anti-stress in the skin means anti-inflammation and aloe vera along with the botanicals, peptides, and minerals that I put in my products help reduce the signs of stressed skin in its tracks!

Chapter 26

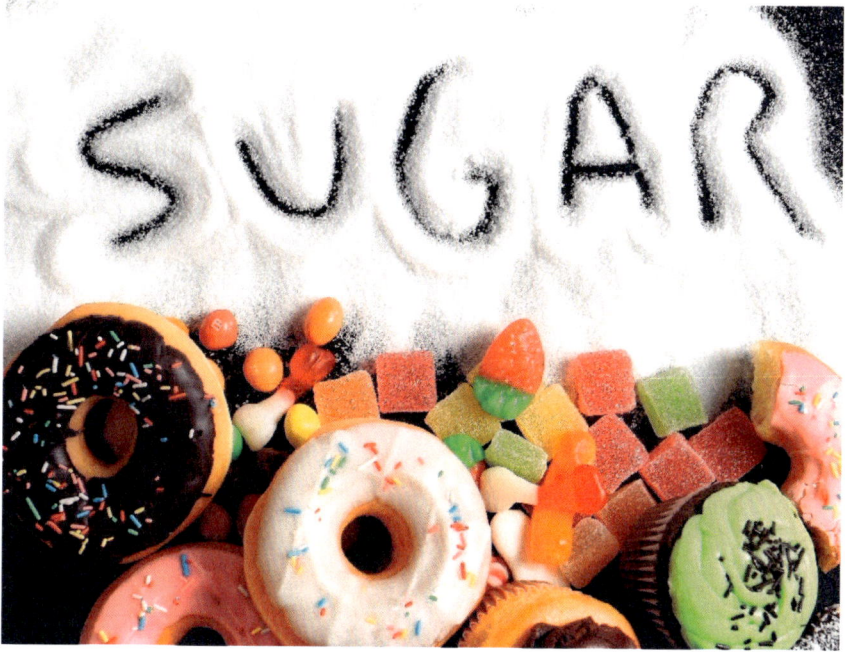

According to the USDA, SUGAR consumption has increased annually since 1982. Sources of SUGAR include cane sugar, beet sugar, high fructose corn syrup, and corn sugar. The World Health Organization now defines too much SUGAR as more than ten percent of an individual's daily caloric intake and recommends only five percent (six teaspoons a day) for better health benefits.

Diabetes has more than doubled since 1980 and obesity has almost tripled since 1960. SUGAR is hidden in bread, pasta, cereals, packaged foods, processed meats, so-called juices and sodas. It is estimated that Americans consume sixty pounds of high fructose corn syrup a year. This was not around in the 60's and as I recall, there were really not a lot of overweight people either. In 1980, one in seven people were obese and six million had diabetes. In 2011, one in three people were obese and nineteen million people had diabetes, with another seven million not diagnosed. A whopping seventy-nine million people had pre-diabetes and unfortunately, the numbers just keeping soaring each year. The link between obesity, SUGAR, and diabetes is clear. For more information on obesity please review the chapter called SIZE MATTERS.

Let's take a closer look at SUGAR. Here is a little SUGAR 101:

- **Glucose** is the primary source of energy for the body as it breaks down carbohydrates, protein and fat by the liver and kidneys. Glucose triggers the release of hormones that make you feel full because eighty percent is used directly by cells and only twenty percent is stored for future use. Also, eighty percent is absorbed by the intestines and only twenty percent by the liver. The body makes glucose from all food sources: carbohydrates (mostly), proteins, and fats.

- **Fructose** (as opposed to glucose) occurs naturally in fruits and vegetables. The problem is not the modest amount of fructose that comes from fruits and sugar-rich vegetables as a part of a balanced diet in which the body has no problem breaking down easily. **The problem comes from high fructose corn syrup.** Its different molecular structure forces the body to use this source of energy in a different way.

  It does not trigger the release of leptin or insulin that controls the appetite by making you feel full. It is converted into glycerol, THE MAIN COMPONENT OF TRIGLYCERIDES which turns into fat formation. One hundred percent of it is processed by the liver increasing the toxic load there. This type of SUGAR raises your triglycerides.

- **Sucrose** is half fructose and half glucose and comes in the form of table sugar, granulated cane sugar, or beet sugar. When you consume this form of sugar, as well as, high fructose corn syrup, your body must first break them down into the most basic components of glucose and fructose before absorption.

The addition of this type of SUGAR to practically every food that is manufactured is overloading the natural digestive process of the body and confusing to the public since they are promoted as 'natural.' **Too much table sugar and high fructose corn syrup cause obesity and diabetes.**

Your pancreas is responsible for producing a hormone called insulin which opens your cells so glucose can get in. The cells use glucose for energy or store for future use. In some cases, cells do not respond properly to insulin, they actually resist it. Since the cells do not want to open up and use the glucose, it builds up in the blood.

Now, the pancreas is freaking out. It still sees all that glucose running around in the blood, so it pumps out more insulin, which causes a build-up of insulin in the blood.

Obviously, this is not good. Beta cells in the pancreas that make insulin eventually wear out. Since no more insulin can be produced to keep glucose in check, pre-diabetes is the result. Pre-diabetes is also known as type 2 diabetes.

- If you have high glucose levels, high triglycerides, high LDL (bad cholesterol), and low HDL, you probably have insulin resistance.

- If you have been diagnosed with pre-diabetes, you probably have insulin resistance.

- If you want to stop insulin resistance, you will have to reduce SUGAR and simple carbs. It's not rocket science.

INSULIN RESISTANCE NOW,
DIABETES TO COME

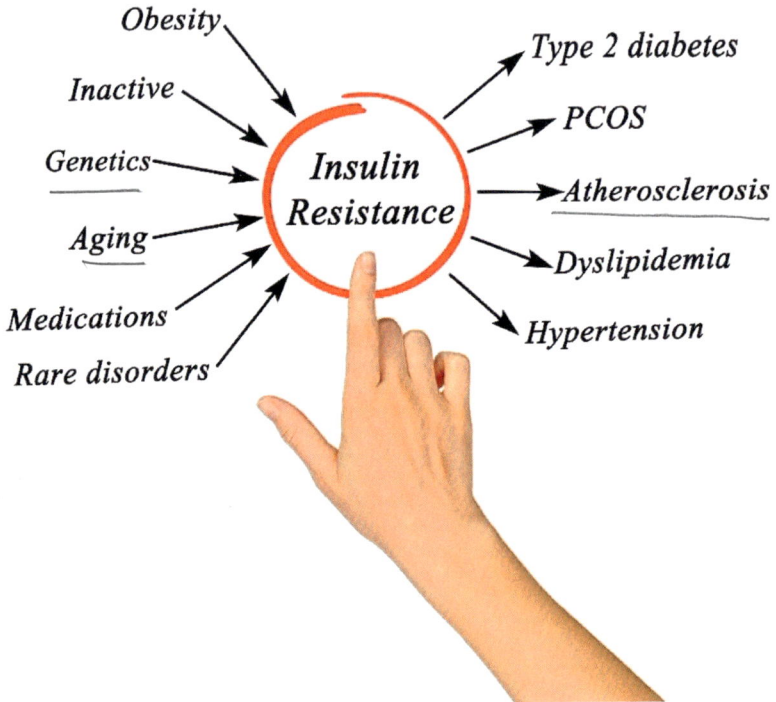

Now numerous scientific studies (America's National Center for Biotechnology Information) show the link of thirty percent increase in developing prostate cancer, forty-four percent in rectal cancer and forty-one percent in pancreatic cancer to increased SUGAR consumption. SUGAR stimulates insulin production which in turn stimulates a hormone called 'insulin-like growth factor' which cancer depends upon for fuel and to grow.

Heart disease is the number one cause of death in America (occurring 15-20 years earlier than the global average) and once again high SUGAR intake is the biggest contributor to increase the rate of this disease. Studies reveal that people who get ten to twenty-four percent of their calories from added SUGAR are thirty percent more likely to die from cardio-vascular disease than those who consume less.

In fact, according to a study done by the University of California in 2012, SUGAR was responsible for over thirty-five million deaths worldwide.

OK, so it is clear that SUGAR makes you fat and sick and apparently, to be blunt, will kill you. Now, what does it do to the skin? There is a process called glycation where SUGAR breaks down and binds with protein molecules including skin collagen and elastin. This overall degradation of the protein that holds your skin together **causes premature aging**. So, if you have a sweet tooth, you will have more wrinkles sooner than you should.

It's time to get serious about this deadly food. Keep track of your daily SUGAR intake. Learn to read labels and look for the SUGAR content. If you see more than 4g do not buy it. If it says high fructose corn syrup don't buy it. Agave nectar, maple syrup and honey are suitable natural sweeteners but should be used sparingly. Stevia and Monk Fruit are great natural substitutes for sweetening drinks and desserts and add no sugar grams (or calories) to your daily count.

By adding more naturally sweet vegetables and fruits you can crowd out your sugar cravings. Carrots, onions, beets, winter squash, sweet potatoes and yams are considered sweet vegetables. Turnips, parsnips, and rutabagas are semi-sweet while red radishes, daikon, green cabbage, burdock and celery root don't taste sweet, but have a similar effect on the body in that they maintain blood SUGAR levels, reduce sweet cravings, and break down animal foods in the body.

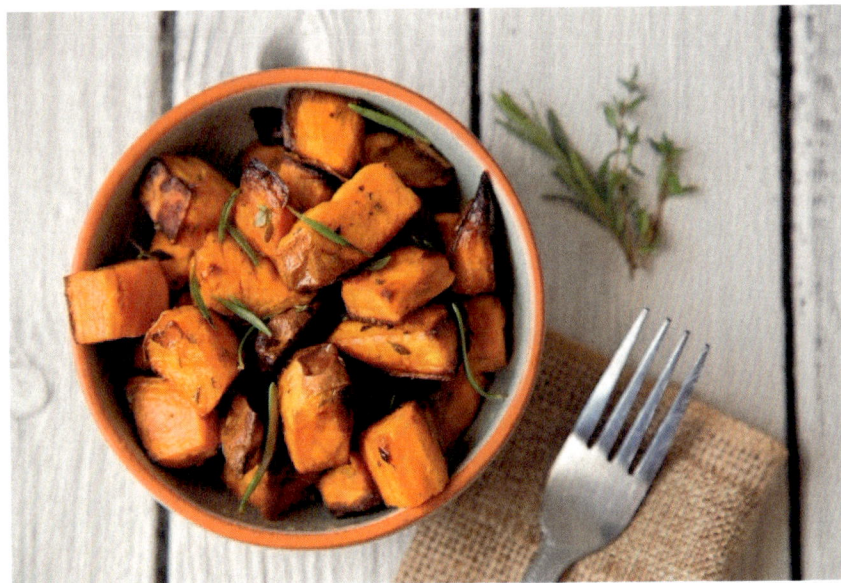

I love to roast most of these in bite size pieces with my favorite herbs and tossed in a little melted coconut oil. Alpha Lipoic Acid, chromium, vanadium, and zinc are excellent supplements to help control blood sugar levels.

If you want to slow down the aging process, you will have to stop eating all those pastries, cakes, cookies, puddings, ice cream, candy bars, fruit-filled yogurt and protein bars. You will also have to read the labels of pre-packaged foods like cereals, crackers, bread, mixes, sauces, and pasta and put them back on the shelf if they contain more than 4g of SUGAR.

If you want to live younger longer, get serious about eliminating this sweet killer!

Just think the way I do: No SUGAR, no wrinkles

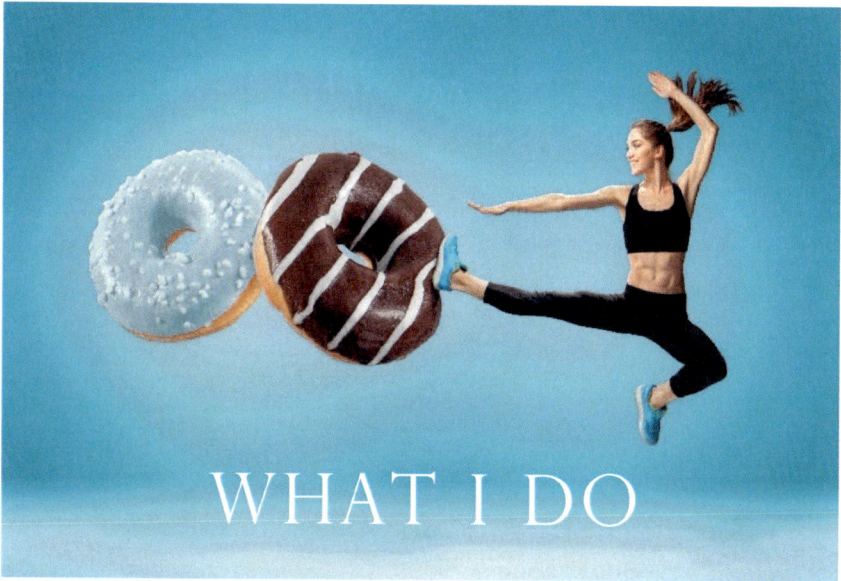

WHAT I DO

1. I read all labels to check the sugar content. If it is more than 4g, I don't buy it with the exception of seventy-two percent dark chocolate bars. The benefits of the chocolate are greater than the sugar content.

2. I make sugar-free, gluten-free desserts with Monk Fruit and stevia. They taste great and conversion rates come on the packaging.

3. As I said earlier, I grill, roast, stir-fry or best of all poach in water all the vegetables I mentioned above with rosemary, garlic, ginger, turmeric, herbs de Provence, chili powder, curry powder, cinnamon, salt, pepper, etc. I try to pair the seasoning with the theme of the rest of the meal.

4. I never drink sodas or fruity drinks. Even most 'real' fruit drinks have too much sugar.

5. I use stevia in my tea, coffee, and smoothies.

6. I order fresh fruit for dessert if available when eating out.

7. I bring stevia packets with me everywhere I go!

8. I don't buy any manufactured products with high fructose corn syrup.

9. For my gluten-free pancakes, I use organic 100% Maple Syrup. It does not affect blood sugar like syrup made with sugar or high fructose corn syrup.

10. I don't eat cakes, donuts, pies, brownies, etc. that seem to be the main course for most church gatherings along with sugary drinks. It is sad that these social functions are serving such unhealthy, disease causing treats. It is my hope that this information finds its way to my fellow brothers and sisters. The *Bible* says: "My people perish for lack of knowledge." Hosea 4:6

Chapter 27

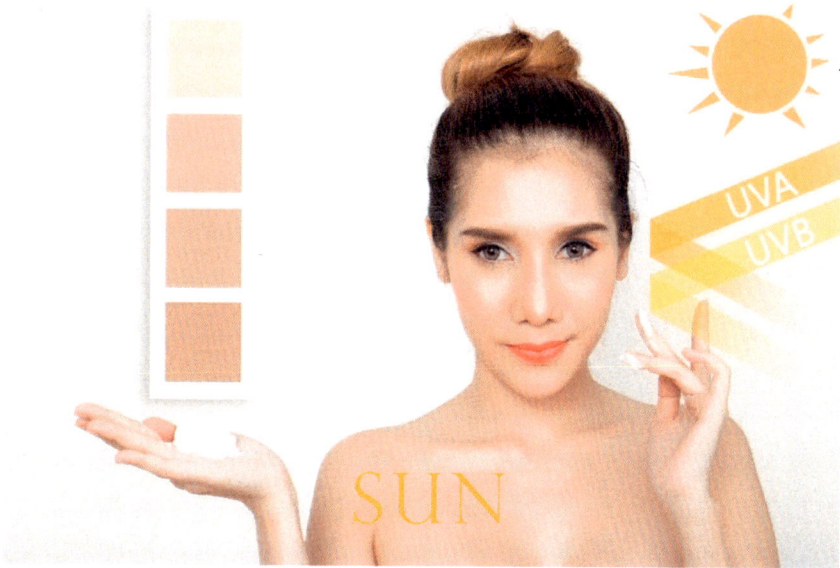

Is the SUN your friend or foe when it comes to aging? Let's examine the possibilities. Only thirty percent of your melanoma risk is tied to genetics and with non-melanoma skin cancers, it's about ten percent.

So, having more than fifty moles and a number of past sunburns makes you more at risk than your family history. If you have had more than five sunburns in your lifetime, then your risk for melanoma has doubled. And just one indoor tanning session before age thirty-five ups your odds of melanoma by seventy-five percent.

Having said all that, the SUN still may be more friend than foe. There is new research done in Norway, England, and the United States by Dr. William Grant and others shattering current SUN myths!

- **Myth #1**: Stay out of the SUN between 10 a.m. and 2 p.m. Turns out, this is the best time to produce vitamin D because the UVB rays are more intense so a shorter exposure time is needed. (Remember UVB rays produce vitamin D). While a lifetime of UVB is linked to squamous cell carcinoma, UVA irradiant and sporadic sun burning causes melanoma.

  Cutaneous malignant melanoma is the most serious skin cancer accounting for three-fourths of all skin cancer deaths. So, avoiding the midday SUN, and thinking all other times are better (so you stay longer), will actually increase your cancer risk, explains Dr. Grant.

- **Myth #2**: The best time for SUN exposure is before 10 a.m. and after 4 p.m. Unfortunately, at this time, the angle of the Sun rays has to penetrate through more atmosphere and the UVB rays (which are shorter than UVA rays) are mostly filtered out. UVA rays, on the other hand, reach right through the atmosphere right to your skin and through the skin's surface causing photo aging, wrinkles, and skin cancer.

- **Myth #3**: Occasional exposure of your face and hands to sunlight is sufficient for obtaining enough vitamin D. Dr. Joseph Mercola explains, "This is miserably inadequate exposure to move vitamin D levels to a healthy range." Shorts, sleeveless tops, and bathing suits are necessary to reveal enough skin to manufacture vitamin D.

- **Myth #4**: Everyone needs around twenty minutes of SUN exposure every day. Apparently, that is correct for light skinned Caucasians. For darkly pigmented skin, it can take three to six times longer to raise Vitamin D levels sufficiently. For each though, longer exposure times are required in the spring, fall and winter.

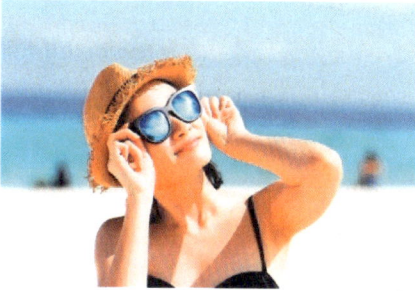

Myth #5: Going out in the SUN will increase your cancer risk. According to Dr. Grant, thirty percent of cancer deaths could be prevented world-wide with higher vitamin D levels.

That is around two hundred thousand lives in the U.S. His research revealed the skin cancer rates of people in higher altitudes such as Iceland were four times higher than in the tropics around the equator. He concluded that there is an anti-cancer protective effect of getting more Vitamin D from regular sun exposure.

- **Myth #6**: Eating vitamin D fortified foods provide enough vitamin D. Optimum vitamin D levels of 2000 IU to 4000 IU will reduce your cancer risk by fifty percent. The average American diet supplies around 250 IU to 350 IU daily, so SUN exposure is essential. Vitamin D is really a steroid hormone (not a regular vitamin) and is best obtained through the SUN. In winter months, have your vitamin D levels tested for proper supplementation. Vitamin D is found naturally in eggs, organ meats, animal fat, cod liver oil, and fish.

What is the take away from these new studies? You need a little midday SUN because you need to manufacture vitamin D. Vitamin D is necessary to prevent cancer. Vitamin D deficiency is also linked to heart disease, autoimmune diseases, infections, bone density, and mental health conditions.

SUN exposure is good, sunburns are bad. If you have darker skin, you will need longer SUN exposure times. Eating the right foods will not give you enough vitamin D.

Repeated and prolonged exposure to UVA rays damage the skin's cellular DNA, making it impossible to repair and rebuild your collagen/elastin fibers that keep your skin plump and smooth.

What about sunscreens? New studies show that chemically derived sunscreens may not be the answer either. They are also creating DNA damage and disrupting hormones. Look for sunscreens made with non-nano zinc or titanium dioxide suggests Dr. Joseph Mercola.

He explains that nano particles could be small enough to penetrate the skin and enter the bloodstream which could have negative side effects as well. In conclusion, he says that zinc and titanium are the best choices for sun protection but still should only be used when going directly into the sun for a prolonged period of time. **That's right; sunscreens should not be used on a daily basis.**

The SUN can be your friend and give you a healthy dose of Vitamin D which is necessary for prevention of many diseases and cancers (colon, ovarian, pancreatic, prostate, and Hodgkin's lymphoma). It produces the feel-good hormone, serotonin that prevents a type of depression called Seasonal Affective Disorder (SAD

The SUN heals certain skin conditions like psoriasis, eczema, jaundice, and thyroiditis. SUN Gazing has been trending for over a decade. NASA studies do show it does have health and anti-aging benefits. Check it out and see if it is right for you.

Know how to make the SUN your friend not your foe if you want to live younger, longer.

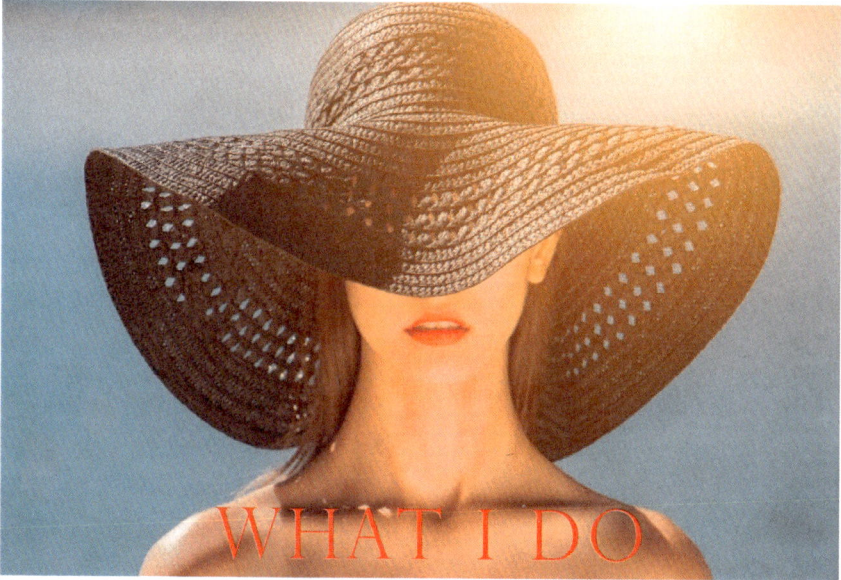
WHAT I DO

1. Whether I am at the pool or at the beach, I stay under an umbrella or covered area when I have had enough sun exposure.

2. I wear hats or sun visors and sun glasses.

3. If I am playing golf or volleyball I use Goddess Garden Organics sunscreen (which I sell also to my clients). I am sure there are other brands. Just look for non-nano zinc and titanium as the active agent, not a bunch of chemicals.

4. I also make my own sunscreen by putting a couple tablespoons of zinc oxide into my Aloe Vera Body Lotion.

5. Another great recipe for all the do-it-yourself types is: ½ cup almond oil with a tsp. red raspberry seed oil and a tsp. carrot seed oil, ¼ cup coconut oil, ¼ cup beeswax (optional), 2 tbsp. shea butter or coconut oil, vanilla extract for fragrance, and 2 tbsp. of non-nano zinc oxide. Combine all ingredients (except zinc) in a glass jar and place in a pot with 2 inches of water. Melt ingredients, add zinc oxide (wear mask), and combine

thoroughly. Stir well   move from heat. Place lid and store in a cool place.

6. If I get too much SUN, I cut open the leaf of an aloe vera plant and spread the gel of the inner leaf over the affected area. (The aloe plant has anti-inflammatory agents that instantly cease pain and activate healing).

7. When on vacation, I bring our pure Aloe Gel for skin healing emergencies.

8. I take Coenzyme Q10 and Astaxanthin supplements daily to help protect my skin from DNA damage..

9. I use my Hello Gorgeous Q10 Booster with MSM to repair sun damage under my Hello Gorgeous PM cream.

10. I take Vitamin D supplements in the winter and when not getting much SUN exposure. (Get tested.)

11. I double up on omega-3s when going to the beach to inhibit inflammation and to increase the time spent out-doors!!

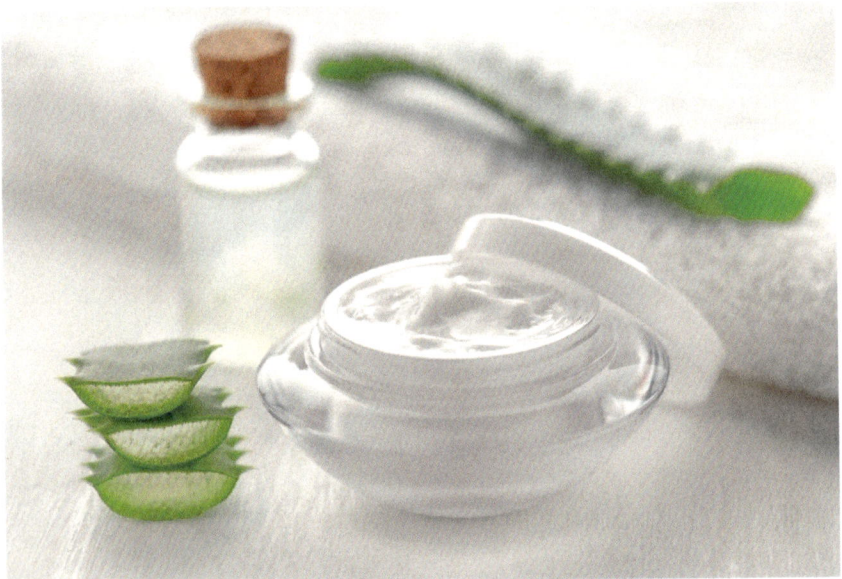

Chapter 28

SWEAT

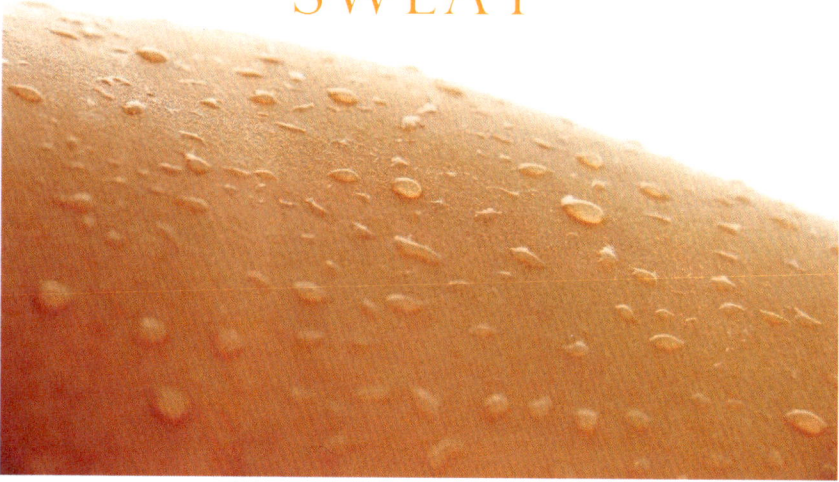

OK, sweating out toxins is a good thing! I'm really talking about **dehydration**, but it didn't start with an 'S' so I had to improvise a little. ☺ I had a doctor on my radio show called: *Health & Beauty Talk,* who told me years ago that all disease was caused by STRESS, MALNUTRITION, and DEHYDRATION. In the book: *Your Body's Many Cries For Water*, the author explains that **"you are not sick, you are thirsty."**

I have addressed the stress and malnutrition, but let's dig a little deeper into dehydration.

Water makes up to eighty-three percent of your blood volume, so it's easy to see why it is important to anti-aging. Your blood carries oxygen and nutrients to tissues through the arterial and capillary system, as well as, carbon dioxide, by-products, and waste products through the venous system ultimately discharging through the lungs, sweat, stool and urine.

All in all, water makes up almost two-thirds of your body mass and through intercellular fluids, unites various organs and systems for critical communication.

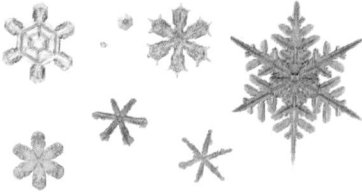

Water 101: Many are unaware that water is actually a liquid crystal, with its' own unique characteristics. Even though water is defined as two parts hydrogen and one-part oxygen, every water molecule is different. Perhaps you have seen the pictures of snowflakes; there are no two snowflakes that are the same. Not only are they unique, water molecules carry information.

A Japanese scientist, Dr. Masaru Emoto, conducted experiments where he spoke to water and then froze it. When he said to the water: "you make me sick," the water crystal formed was a chaotic structure much like a cancerous tumor. When he spoke the word "love" to the water and froze it, it became a beautiful geometric crystalline structure.

Another experiment with the same water was with two names: Adolf Hitler and Mother Theresa. The same water molecule when frozen became two distinct formations with one being chaotic and the other a perfect crystalline structure. This brings new meaning to the *Bible* scripture in Proverbs 18:21 that says, "Death and life are in the power of the tongue, and they that love it shall eat the fruit thereof."

Water is a source of energy that carries information to your body's self-healing forces to activate regeneration. I'm sure you have heard of the thousands of healings from 'holy' springs around the world. In fact, these waters have been tested and have been found to be different from typical drinking waters. Natural spring waters

defy gravity and make their way to the surface from thousands of feet down into the earth's belly.

The book, *Water and Salt, The Essence of Life,* explains that the water has matured below and carries sufficient forces of levitation to make its way to the surface. While deep below the surface it absorbs the electromagnetic field of the earth which is 7.83 Hertz. **Our body has the same frequency pattern as a water molecule.**

The book goes on to explain that natural spring water is better able to replenish what your body is missing (the energy deficit) when you are ill and out of balance. Now you know why you are told to drink plenty of fluids when you are sick. Actually, the doctor should tell you to only drink natural spring water!

Scientists believe the overall health benefits of natural spring water come from its perfectly structured molecules capable of creating an overall information pattern. I'm sure you have heard of the 'healing' spring water of Fatima and Lourdes.

They also have a natural pH of 7.5 (slightly alkaline which keeps the body from getting too acidic which is where disease strives). Many spring waters contain a high amount of colloidal silica known for skin, nails, bone, and hair restoration and are also known to improve brain function.

When choosing natural spring water, it is important to trust the source since it could be recycled tap water. I love the taste of spring water like Fiji and others. Untreated, natural spring water clearly tastes different.

Without water, your cells begin to die. You need water to regulate body temperature, remove wastes, and bring nutrients to cells.

If you are dehydrated, nothing in your body is functioning properly and aging is accelerated.

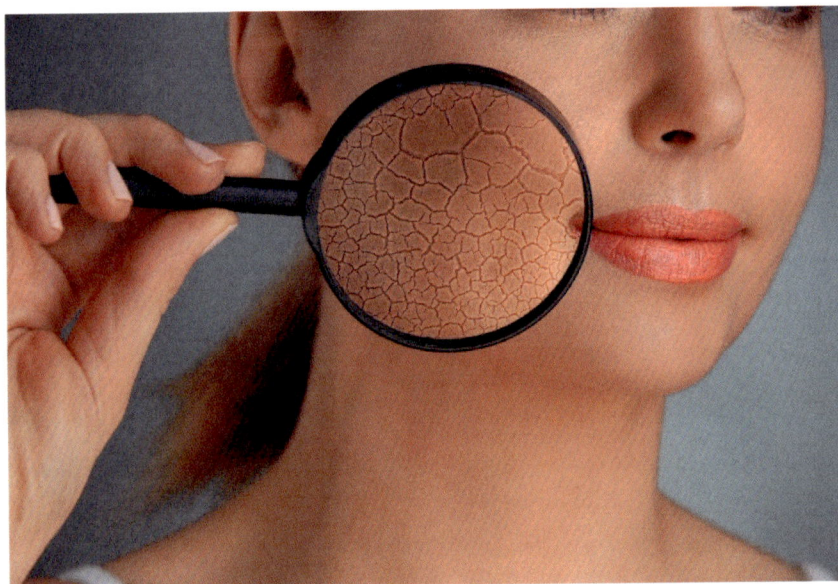

Men need to drink around three liters (thirteen cups) a day and women need two liters (nine cups) a day. Some health coaches suggest half your body weight in ounces. Obviously, if you have an active lifestyle and SWEAT a lot, you will need much more. Cokes and coffee cannot replace water intake, but green or white tea can replace some of it.

Let's move on to my favorite section, what happens to your face! **There is actually a condition called TEWL**. It stands for trans-epidermal water loss and is basically dehydrated skin. As one gets older, the skin integrity loosens, and a type of evaporation occurs. Also, as one ages, the production of hyaluronic acid (HA) slows down and almost comes to a screeching halt. What is HA?

It's that wonderful substance inside the cell that attracts moisture up to one thousand times its molecular weight. It is THE super humectant. HA is abundant in skin cells in your youth and is what makes children's skin look so plump and smooth. By the age of forty, the human body slows down production of this magical substance. It now must be obtained through the skin with topical application or from the inside from food. **Without hydration your skin shrinks, shrivels, and screams: "I'm old."**

So, what do you do? Just drinking more water doesn't help the outer layers of skin as much as eating more fruits and vegetables will. Melons, cucumbers, citrus fruit and green leafy vegetables are best for skin re-hydration. To eat more HA, add more root vegetables, chicken and beef broths, leafy greens, and fermented soy products. Studies show even red wine will increase the amount of hyaluronic production.

Use a good hydrating skin care system faithfully. Unfortunately, most skin care products are about eighty percent water and your skin is basically waterproof. That is why you don't soak up all the water in the bath tub or the swimming pool and blow up like a 'floaty.' In fact, water like that can dehydrate you. Ever noticed how your fingers shrivel up when you are in the pool or hot tub a long time? Of course, I recommend HG aloe-based products.

I hope you can see that not all water is equal. Concerns of chemically-washed city water, pesticide run off and toxin contamination have led consumers to buy bottled water. Did you know that forty-five percent of all bottled water is re-purposed municipal water? I'm happy to see that the sixteen-billion-dollar water industry of 2016 surpassed the SODA as the number one drink sold in the U.S., but like I said, not all water is equal. In my opinion, the best water is naturally sourced spring water and my favorite is Fiji.

If you want to stay younger longer, you will have to avoid dehydration and ***drink more natural spring water***

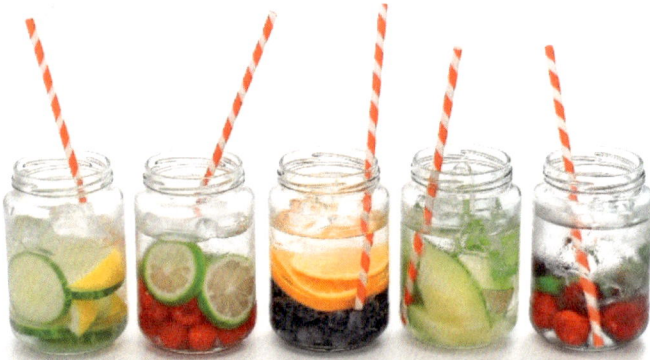

WHAT I DO

1. I eat lots of salads because they are loaded with H_2O. I collect salad recipes because you can only eat so much lettuce and tomatoes.

2. I use filtered water for cooking and drink Fiji water throughout the day.

3. I make fun spa water (place water in a glass container with colorful fruit and herbs) to serve at meals.

4. I love to cook a variety of "colors" for each meal and that usually means a few root vegetables baked in the oven, poached in water, or stir-fried.

5. When I cook rice, quinoa, or gluten-free noodles, I use beef or chicken broth instead of plain water to add more nutritional elements.

6. I add collagen with hyaluronic to my morning smoothies or just mix a quick batch with almond milk.

7. I do drink red wine, the fact that it helps me make HA is my new excuse!

8. I never skip my AM or PM skin care regimens. This helps prevent TEWL. If you live in colder climates, you may need an extra layer of moisturizer for added protection. Coconut oil is a great addition on top of body moisturizers, but use only occasionally on the face at it will clog pores.

9. I also wear makeup every day. I won't even go to the mailbox without makeup. (Just kidding.) Seriously, makeup is another way to prevent TEWL.

10. Humectants are very important in a skin care system to help prevent TEWL. My Hello Gorgeous creams, serums, and toners are around seventy-five percent aloe vera which is one of nature's finest humectants (a substance that attracts and holds moisture). I've also included HA and other phyto-humectants like glycerin, sodium PCA, sorbitol, allantoin, and glycosaminoglycans. My moisturizers really do moisturize!

11. What about HA injections? I have had a few in scars on my face and they are almost gone now. They also can add volume to cheeks and lips. I may try that too! It seems there are no harmful side effects and it is a lot cheaper than a face lift.

Chapter 29

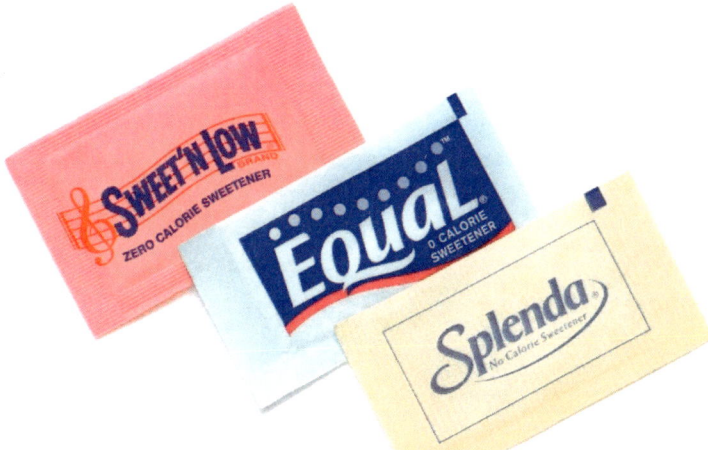

SWEETENERS

It is so necessary to also talk about artificial SWEETENERS. This is another 'S' Word that is sabotaging your health and longevity. **Imagine for a moment a person wearing a white lab coat and mask standing in a laboratory creating a concoction of odorless crystal powder.** Almost sounds criminal, and probably should be. Here are some of the mad-scientist's creations:

- Aspartame (Equal, Nutra Sweet, Natra Taste Blue)

- Sucralose (Splenda)

- Acesulfame K (ACE K, Sunette, Equal Spoonful, Sweet One, Sweet'n Safe)

- Saccharine (Sweet 'N Low, Sweet Trim)

If these non-nutritive powders were so effective and non-harmful, why has obesity and diabetes skyrocketed since the 1950s when they were first introduced into the food market?

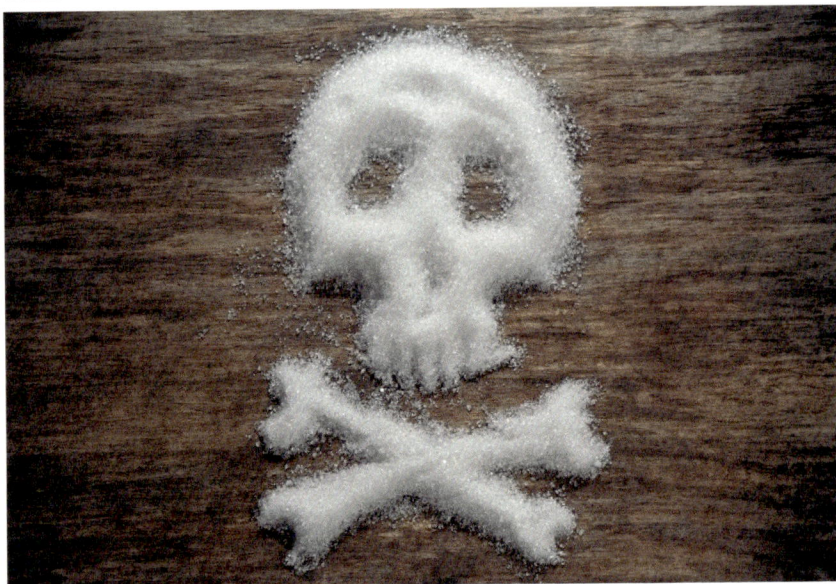

Studies that proclaim their safety are usually performed with quantities far less than the current consumption.

Aspartame is comprised of phenylalanine, aspartic acid, and methanol (sounds delicious) and is currently used in six thousand consumer foods and drinks and over five hundred prescription drugs. Sucralose is a chlorinated derivative of sugar (chlorine is toxic) discovered when developing a new pesticide. Acesulfame K (ACE, ACE K) is comprised of a potassium salt that contains methylene chloride. Saccharin is a sulfa-based sweetener which once required a warning label because it caused cancer in animal studies, but the FDA has removed that warning.

The Journal of Toxicology and Environmental Health found that a toxic compound called chloropropanols, forms when cooking with sucralose. *The American Journal of Industrial Medicine* has recently published a study calling for a "re-evaluation" of sucralose that "must be considered an urgent matter of public health."

The AARP followed 264,000 U.S. adults over fifty for ten years to evaluate their diet and health. The *Environmental Health Perspectives* review found that those who drank more than four diet sodas or artificially sweetened beverages had a **thirty percent higher risk of depression.**

The Public Library of Science's journal, *PLOS ONE,* published research that confirmed regularly consuming artificially sweetened beverages is associated with:

- Metabolic Syndrome
- Abdominal Obesity
- Insulin Resistance
- Impaired Glucose Intolerance
- Abnormally Elevated Fats in The Blood
- High Blood Pressure
- Pre-Diabetes

Research from Ramazzine Institute in Bologna, Italy, has linked Splenda to cancer, specifically leukemia. Splenda is found in over four thousand five hundred products. Even more stunning, some of these SWEETENERS are linked to retinol damage, brain damage, DNA damage, and birth defects.

Obviously, these laboratory concoctions are not good for your skin. Consuming non-nutritive substances won't nourish any cell in your body and malnutrition shows up first on the skin as a warning of what is going on inside your body.

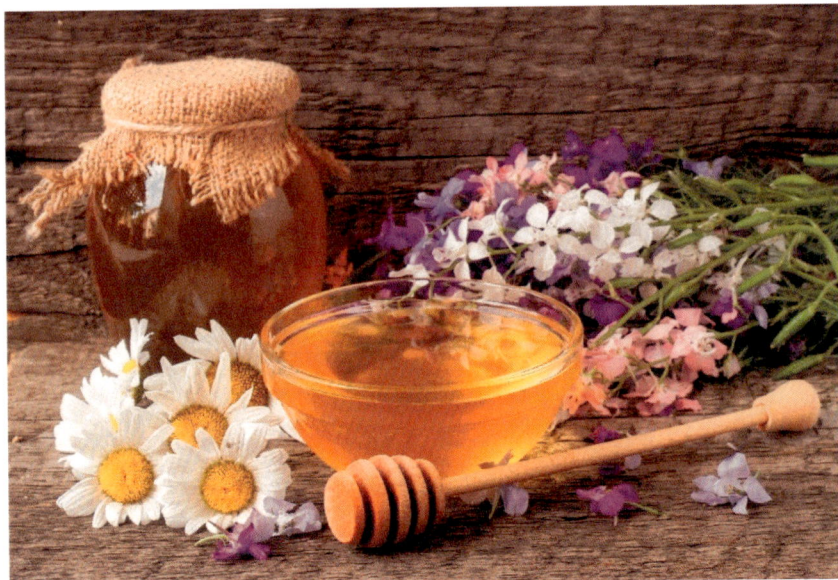

The chapter on SODAS reveals even more harmful diseases caused by DIET SODAS made with these toxic SWEETENERS. Learn to love all-natural sweeteners like maple syrup, monk fruit, stevia, fruit purees, and raw honey. Follow the suggestions I made under SUGAR. Add vanilla, cocoa, licorice, nutmeg, and cinnamon to root vegetables and other foods to enhance their sweetness.

Look for cookbooks featuring all-natural sweeteners. Keep stevia packets in your purse or car so you won't be tempted to reach for the 'blue and pink' packets on the restaurant table. Exercising on a regular basis will significantly reduce food and sugar cravings.

Is consuming this FAKE FOOD worth the risk? If you want to slow down the aging process, you must stop consuming artificial SWEETENERS.

If you want to live younger longer, you must EAT NATURAL SWEETENERS!

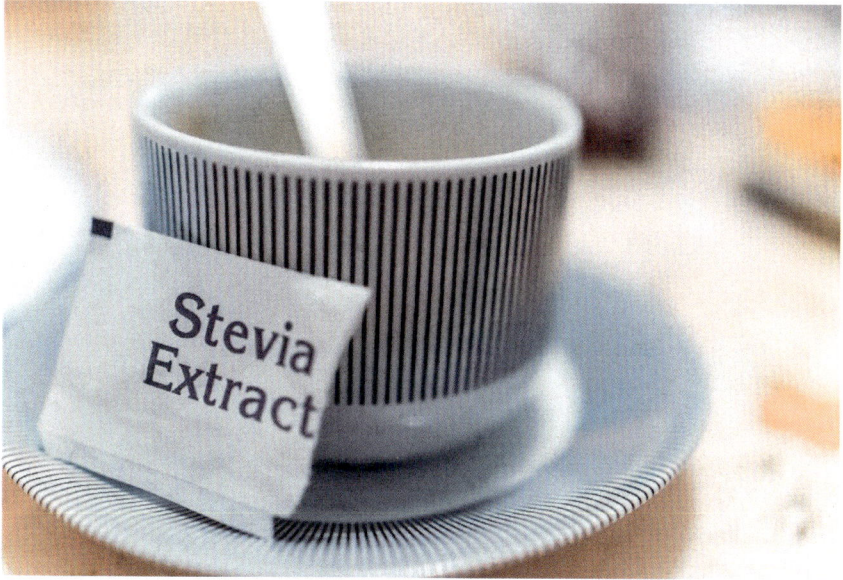

1. I don't buy anything that says 'sugar-free.'

2. I use stevia to sweeten my tea, smoothies, and coffee.

3. I keep stevia packets in my purse.

4. I make desserts with honey, maple syrup, Monk Fruit, and stevia.

5. I read all labels to look for 'hidden sweeteners.'

6. I drink water with lemon because it reduces the cravings for sweets.

7. I eat fermented vegetables to reduce the cravings for sweets.

8. I do some form of exercise every day.

FINAL THOUGHTS
SUCCESSFULLY AGING

Aging successfully means avoiding a few S WORDS literally! I've always thought aging gracefully was just a way of saying that this is the way it is, so get over it. The Institute On Aging, and the *Bible* for that matter, say we are supposed to live successfully for one hundred and twenty years. Why aren't we?

Every ten years we replace every cell in our body, so why aren't we just getting better and better? Because those darn 'S Words' are subtly sabotaging our chances.

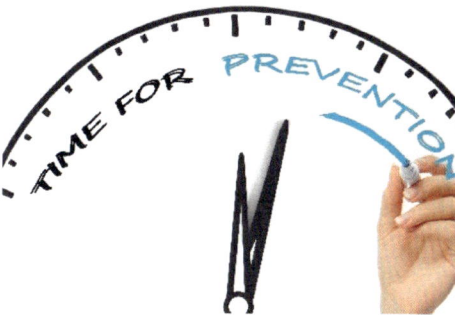

Now that you are aware of these aging culprits you can choose to live and live life more abundantly. But remember, information alone is not transformation. Dr. D. L. Katz says, "Life and death, knowledge and power: why knowing what matters isn't what's the matter." Aristotle said it something like this, "You are what you repeatedly do. Excellence therefore, is not an act but a habit."

I like to put it like this, "You are what you eat, think, and do." It's all up to you my beautiful friend. Aging doesn't mean you MUST get OLD and SICK.

Let's live like we love it and feel young while we are doing it!

AGE SUCCESSFULLY AND LIVE YOUNGER LONGER!

BOOMER BEAUTY E-BOOK

HOW DO YOU WANT TO LOOK NOW?

I have gathered a few common-sense beauty tips for all the boomers that are easy to do or not do. The image coach and makeup artist in me just couldn't sit by without giving a few tips on how to LOOK YOUNGER NOW!

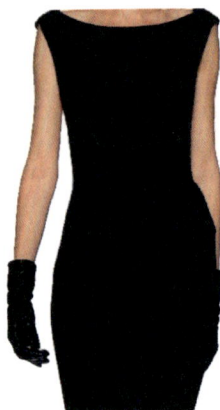

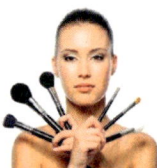

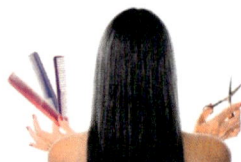

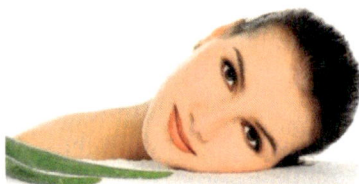

I've included WARDROBE, SKIN CARE, MAKEUP, AND HAIR tips to help you navigate the senior world in style. Who doesn't want to look better, slimmer, and today?

Remember only a confident woman can inspire others with compliments and encouragement. Make your boomer years your best years!

Say "Hello Gorgeous" to someone today and see their face light up with a giant smile! Remember, smiles are contagious!

Request your FREE E-BOOK: *LOOK YOUNGER NOW*, from orders@hellogorgeous.com.

53827437R00122

Made in the USA
Columbia, SC
22 March 2019